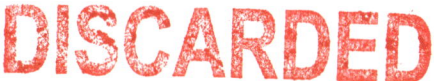

FAMILY DIVERSITY AND FAMILY POLICY:
Strengthening Families for America's Children

OUTREACH SCHOLARSHIP

Editor:

Richard M. Lerner
Tufts University
Medford, Massachusetts, U.S.A.

Forthcoming book in the series:

Ralston, P., Lerner, R., Mullis, A., Simerly, C., and Murray, J.
*Social Change, Public Policy, and Community Collaboration:
Training Human Development Professionals for the 21st Century*

FAMILY DIVERSITY AND FAMILY POLICY:
Strengthening Families for America's Children

Richard M. Lerner
Tufts University

Elizabeth E. Sparks
Boston College

and

Laurie D. McCubbin
University of Wisconsin-Madison

OUTREACH SCHOLARSHIP
Series Editor: Richard M. Lerner

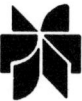

KLUWER ACADEMIC PUBLISHERS
Boston / Dordrecht / London

Distributors for North, Central and South America:
Kluwer Academic Publishers
101 Philip Drive
Assinippi Park
Norwell, Massachusetts 02061 USA
Telephone (781) 871-6600
Fax (781) 871-6528
E-Mail <kluwer@wkap.com>

Distributors for all other countries:
Kluwer Academic Publishers Group
Distribution Centre
Post Office Box 322
3300 AH Dordrecht, THE NETHERLANDS
Telephone 31 78 6392 392
Fax 31 78 6546 474
E-Mail <services@wkap.nl>

 Electronic Services <http://www.wkap.nl>

Library of Congress Cataloging-in-Publication Data
Lerner, Richard M.
    Family diversity and family policy: strengthening families for
  America's children / Richard M. Lerner, Elizabeth E. Sparks, and
  Laurie D. McCubbin.
       p.   cm. -- (Outreach scholarship)
  Includes bibliographical references and indexes.
  ISBN 0-7923-8612-4 (alk. paper)
  1. Family -- United States. 2. Family policy -- United States.
3. Pluralism (Social sciences) -- United States. I. Sparks,
Elizabeth E. II. McCubbin, Laurie D. III. Title. IV. Series.
HQ535.L39   1999
306.85'0973--dc21   99-40718
                                                               CIP

Copyright © 1999 by Kluwer Academic Publishers

All rights reserved. No part of this publication may be reproduced, stored in a retrieval system or transmitted in any form or by any means, mechanical, photo-copying, recording, or otherwise, without the prior written permission of the publisher, Kluwer Academic Publishers, 101 Philip Drive, Assinippi Park, Norwell, Massachusetts 02061
Printed on acid-free paper.
Printed in the United States of America

CONTENTS

Foreword
    Karen Bogenschneider   vii

Foreword
    Harriette Pipes McAdoo   xiii

Preface   xvii

1. THE FAMILY: HISTORICAL AND CONTEMPORARY PERSPECTIVES   1

2. CHILD POVERTY WITHIN THE ECOLOGY OF AMERICA'S FAMILIES   13

3. DEVELOPMENTAL CONTEXTUALISM AND THE DEVELOPMENTAL SYSTEMS PERSPECTIVE   25

4. ENGAGING PUBLIC POLICY: THE SUBSTANTIVE IMPORTANCE OF DIVERSITY   43

5. THE PARENTING OF ADOLESCENTS AND ADOLESCENTS AS PARENTS   61

6. THE IMPORTANCE OF DIVERSITY IN WELFARE REFORM   79

7. TOWARD THE DEVELOPMENT OF A NATIONAL YOUTH POLICY   109

8. IMPLICATIONS FOR POLICY DESIGN, DELIVERY, AND EVALUATION   127

References   141

Name Index   157

Subject Index   163

FOREWORD

Karen Bogenschneider
University of Wisconsin-Madison

The most important word in the title of this book may be the "and," which links family diversity and family policy. If one could map the cutting-edge ideas of the 1990s, family diversity and family policy undoubtedly would be prominent streams of thought, each gaining momentum but flowing primarily in parallel courses with few junctures. With some notable exceptions, family diversity and family policy have not been linked as often as they could have been or as well as they should have been, especially in light of the significance these linkages have for policymakers, practitioners, and academics alike.

For example, policymakers often are faced with the extraordinarily difficult task of developing a single coherent family policy that must address the multiple needs of diverse families. Practitioners sometimes disseminate boilerplate programs and practices to the families they serve, amidst doubts that they apply equally well to all. Similarly, in academia, the curriculum guides of many departments of human development and family studies map out separate courses in family diversity and family policy, which leaves the student in the unenviable position of trying to integrate these two disparate streams of thought, a daunting task for even the mature scholar.

This book brings to the fore the challenge of integrating family diversity and family policy, two front-burner issues that are typically conceptualized, discussed, and acted upon in isolation from each other. The authors present demographic data that empirically justify integrating family diversity and family policy, and a theoretical framework that provides a conceptual rationale for this integration. I offer enthusiastic support for emphasizing family diversity in policymaking but also a cautionary note about the unexpected consequences that could result if this emphasis is not strategically pursued. Many of my observations are based on my experiences organizing Family Impact Seminars for state policymakers in Wisconsin since 1993. This series of objective, nonpartisan seminars and briefing reports aims to bring a family focus to policymaking, just as economic and environmental considerations have become standard fare in policy debate (Bogenschneider, 1995).

PROVIDING DEMOGRAPHIC DATA TO SUPPORT AN INTEGRATION OF FAMILY DIVERSITY AND FAMILY POLICY

If the goal of policy is to determine "what ought to be," policies are more apt to be effective if grounded in an accurate assessment of "what is" (Seeley, 1985). This book provides an impressive array of data on what families are like today, and also from whence they have come.

Based on my experience in Wisconsin conducting seminars for state policymakers (Bogenschneider, 1995), legislators desire solid data to guide policymaking. Before launching our first seminar, the advisory committee developed several brief descriptions of potential seminar topics. To our surprise, the legislators selected none of the topics we had identified, but instead asked for demographic data on Wisconsin families—their structure, ethnicity, and living arrangements. This book provides the demographic data policymakers desire, such as those describing the silent revolution of maternal employment, the demographic explosion of single parenthood, the kaleidoscope of family forms, the unprecedented levels of divorce, the advent of cohabiting and stepparent families, and the reemergence of widespread child poverty with its disproportionate concentration among racial/ethnic minorities. This book provides a seedbed of information that family professionals can use to prepare policy briefs on the changing landscape of American families.

ADVANCING A THEORETICAL FRAMEWORK FOR INTEGRATING FAMILY DIVERSITY AND FAMILY POLICY

The book takes the important step of advancing a theoretical framework—developmental contextualism—for integrating family diversity and family policy. Tenets of this theory have the potential to shape academic research and to guide the development of policies and programs in several ways, three of which will be articulated here. First, developmental contextualism provides a rationale for emphasizing diversity in policy, practice, and research through its assertion that human development is a dynamic, reciprocal process that occurs when individuals interact with multiple contexts and, therefore, is not necessarily generalizable across diverse people and diverse contexts. Applied to policy, the theory suggests that policymakers continually need to ask and be prompted to ask diversity questions. For example, would different types of welfare recipients benefit from different policy responses? Applied to practice, developmental contextualism would guide program staff to question whether their methods and practices apply generically to all the families in their programs. Applied to research, the theory suggests that researchers track the effectiveness of policies and programs for different types of families. This form of applied scholarship has obvious relevance for practice, but also can inform basic research by testing how sensitive the theories that drive program design and delivery are to family diversity.

Second, the integrative, relational emphases of developmental contextualism provide a rationale for a family focus in policymaking in contrast to the individualistic perspective that has historically pervaded policymaking in this country. Extrapolating from the theory that development involves changes in relationships, the authors contend that policies should focus on the relationship between an individual and the context, not on the individual per se. For the purposes of family policy, the family context is central, but this does not negate the influence other contexts such as peer, school, and community settings have on families and the individuals in them. Some readers might argue that a notable portion of the data that permeate the book emphasizes individual outcomes, thereby contradicting the book's focus on family policy. Instead, I contend that individual data are often needed to document social problems, but that policy responses frequently need to move beyond the individual to the family realm. A number of studies indicate that our programs and policies would be more effective if, instead of ignoring or superseding families, they took into account their impact on family well-being, specifically, family stability, family relationships, and the ability of family members to carry out their responsibilities (Bogenschneider, in press).

As an example, much of the debate on welfare reform has been individually focused, exploring ways to enhance parents' breadwinning capacity and their ability to achieve self-sufficiency through work. Yet the convincing data in this book on the devastating consequences of poverty and welfare receipt on child well-being document the need for a family focus in welfare reform. Family-sensitive policymaking would broaden the emphasis from parents' breadwinning potential to their caregiving capacity, specifically, their ability to support their children's development into competent caring adults. As Barbara Blum (1992) has warned, if welfare reform does not pay attention to children's basic needs and chances for future prosperity, our investment in parents' self-sufficiency may well be squandered.

Finally, the depth and detail of developmental contextualism will appeal to academics, but the authors also describe the theory in terminology that the less theoretically sophisticated can understand. For example, they urge caution about "one size fits all" policies, warning that policies suitable for a particular racial/ethnic group, social class, or community "may be irrelevant, unsuited, or even damaging to families with other characteristics of diversity" (p. 129). This terminology brings to mind one of Madison Avenue's greatest hoaxes, the garment that fits all sizes. For policies as for garments, the fit may be too loose and relaxed for some, too tight and constraining for others. Similarly, the authors suggest a "goodness of fit" between a particular program or policy and the group it intends to benefit, much like garment manufacturers have developed separate lines for petite, tall, and large consumers. We have learned from our experiences with the Wisconsin Family Impact Seminars that providing these visual, tangible frames of reference has the potential to reframe the terms of the policy debate by helping policymakers conceptualize complex issues and explain them to colleagues and constituents. For example, one Family Impact Seminar speaker compared the development of violent juvenile crime to the growth of a vile weed, an analogy a state senator used in a floor debate.

CAUTIONS ABOUT STRATEGICALLY INTEGRATING FAMILY DIVERSITY AND FAMILY POLICY

Promoting more diversity-sensitive research and practice, although arguably an important quest, can have unexpected and unintended consequences if not pursued strategically (see Bogenschneider, 1997). The challenge is knowing when to emphasize how families are different and when to emphasize how they are similar. Understanding the differences in families is a first step in developing effective family policies, but not the only step. Finding commonalities—those processes and practices that cut across race, ethnicity, family structure, education, or gender—is particularly important for policy purposes for a few reasons.

First, if our policy efforts focus too extensively on family diversity, the inherent complexity of designing programs tailored precisely to these diversities can evoke pessimism and choke off meaningful response. Perhaps more importantly, the most widespread and long-term social policies have focused on similarities, such as those between the advantaged and the disadvantaged. According to Wilson (1997), universal programs not targeted to a particular group are less stigmatizing and more apt to generate ongoing political support. In a historical overview of social policies in the United States, Skocpol (1996) concurred that some of the most successful programs delivered benefits to different segments of the population such as the poor and the middle class through the same policy rubric. As examples, Social Security, Medicare, veteran's benefits, and universal public education deliver slightly more services to the economically disadvantaged but also provide a range of services to beneficiaries, irrespective of income.

Importantly, Wilson (1987) did not propose eliminating race-specific or means-tested programs, but suggested instead that they be considered under the umbrella of a more comprehensive universal program. For example, as the authors of this volume point out on page 20, the preferred mode of child care among Mexican Americans is care by relatives. Although Mexican Americans may lack the political muscle to generate support for relative care among state and federal policymakers, they can join with other activists in support of child care legislation that allows for relative care as one of several strategies in a comprehensive initiative. Emphasizing the common interests of families on issues like child care can unite diverse families and broaden the political support needed for enactment and continuation of family-focused policies. Thus, drawing from the scholarly literature, understanding how families are different is essential to designing effective policies; yet recognizing how families are similar enhances the prospects that policies will muster widespread, sustainable support. The fate of a family agenda hinges on the feasibility of pulling together coalitions that transcend class and race (Skocpol & Greenberg, 1997) to promote "common solutions to shared problems" (Wilson, 1997, p. 77).

Similarly, in a recent public agenda survey (1998), citizens expressed reservations about a narrow or exclusive focus on the differences among families without a companion emphasis on their similarities. An opinion poll sponsored by the Thomas B. Fordham Foundation, the American Federation of Teachers, and the

National Education Association surveyed 801 parents in a national random sample. Oversampling in some categories yielded 203 Hispanics, 198 African Americans, and 200 who were foreign born. Almost 9 out of 10 of those surveyed believed in equal opportunity regardless of race, religion, or sex, and 7 out of 10 believed intolerance is the mark of a "bad" American citizen. Yet, despite this respect for diversity, almost 9 out of 10 believed that too much attention is paid to "what separates different ethnic and racial groups and not enough to what they have in common." Although acknowledging that America does not always live up to its ideals, the majority of respondents (84%) believed that the "United States is a unique country that stands for something special in the world."

Echoing these sentiments, Aldous (1991) once said that no other country in the world has ever brought in such a variety of diverse people and tried to make them equal. In her words, "We've come a long way, but it's a tough act to accomplish." The road is tough to travel because few junctures connect "what is" (i.e., a nation of incredibly diverse families) and "what ought to be" (i.e., family policies sensitive to this diversity). The toughness of the task, however, is overshadowed by its fundamental importance to children and families and, thus, to the future of science, policy, and practice.

REFERENCES

Aldous, J. (Discussant). (1991). *Preventing poverty: Possible lessons and imports from Europe and Japan?* Session at the annual meeting of the National Council on Family Relations, Denver, CO.

Blum, B. B. (1992). Preface. In S. Smith, S. Blank, & R. Collins (Eds.), *Pathways to self-sufficiency for two generations: Designing welfare-to-work programs that benefit children and strengthen families* (pp. 1-2). New York: Foundation for Child Development.

Bogenschneider, K. (1995). Roles for professionals in building family policy: A case study of state family impact seminars. *Family Relations, 44*(1), 5-12.

Bogenschneider, K. (1997, August). Parents involvement in the schooling of their adolescents: A proximal process with transcontextual validity. *Journal of Marriage and the Family, 59*, 718-733.

Bogenschneider, K. (in press). Promoting a family perspective in policymaking with state family impact seminars. In W. Dumon (Ed.), *Family policy* (Proceedings of an expert meeting on family impact), Leuven, Belgium.

Public Agenda. (1998). Available: <http://www.publicagenda.org/thankful/thankful.html>.

Seeley, D. (1985). *Education through partnership.* Washington DC: American Enterprise Institute.

Skocpol, T. (1996, November). *The missing middle working parents in U.S. democracy and social policy.* Paper presented at the annual meeting of the National Council on Family Relations, Kansas City, MO.

Skocpol, T., & Greenberg, S. B. (1997). A politics for our times. In S. B. Greenberg & T. Skocpol (Eds.), *The new majority: Toward a popular progressive politics* (pp. 104-129). New Haven, CT: Yale University Press.

Wilson, W. J. (1987). *The truly disadvantaged: The inner city, the underclass, and public policy.* Chicago: University of Chicago Press.

Wilson, W. J. (1997). The new social inequity and affirmative opportunity. In S. B. Greenberg & T. Skocpol (Eds.), *The new majority: Toward a popular progressive politics* (pp. 57-77). New Haven, CT: Yale University Press.

FOREWORD

Harriette Pipes McAdoo
Michigan State University

The cultural and temporal contexts of families must be given more serious scholarly attention. The diversity that is discussed in this book goes beyond the usual examination found in books on family policies that only talk about a commitment to diversity but then go on to the discussion as if true diversity did not really exists. Lerner, Sparks, and McCubbin's excellent explanation of diversity states that diversity is far-ranging and it is found in many different people. The fact is that the presently held developmental theories continue to have a truncated view of the world. They tend to focus only on the European American family. But even those families have changed, as is highlighted in many sections of this book. The diversity that is found within and between groups still tends to not be incorporated into our theories of development. There are insidious patterns, as Bronfenbrenner (1979) and Elder, Modell, and Parke (1993) noted, of ignoring the variations that exists within and across the context of ecological setting. One cannot assume that the generally accepted rules of development will apply to all children and families. The rules of development will have to expand to incorporate the wider definition of families who are from many contextual settings.

Cultural organizations do facilitate the enculturation of the traditional cultural groups. Our various groups are growing in size and intensity. Many of the traditional stereotypes will need to be challenged and are being changed by the children who are now being born. The blending of many groups is being increased because of the increases of immigrations, cross-racial pairings, and ethnic intermarriage. We are developing into a society that is much unlike the one that we now know and have ever known. The newer modalities will be generated from the existing cultures that already exist.

The proportion of youth within the population, in contrast to the growing segment of elderly, is a serious concern. As fewer new workers are well prepared to support the retirement of their elders, we will see an increasing alienation between these age cohorts within our society. The fact that the majority of these youth will be of color or from "minority" status groups is again a serious predicament. If the new and growing segment of the younger population is not provided the education and job training that are essential because of latent ethnic, racial, and gender restrictions, and isolation, the productivity of the entire country will decline. It can be predicted that the growing disparity of resources between these groups could eventually lead to chaos. It is imperative that we implement the adoption of culture-sensitive developmental contextual theories.

The insistence of concentration upon only the most problematic families will lead to inaccurate pictures of the everyday lives of these families, youth, and children, particularly when they are of color. The rich context of families, their social, economic, parental gender configuration, and geographical locations in this country must be taken into account.

Ethnic pride and neighborhood control of organizations must be enhanced by researchers and outreach workers. The concept of the individuality of people has led to the recognition that "one size does not fit all." The question is how much diversity should be taken into account as policies are formulated? How much should the cultural differences or the commonalties be treated in order to not fall victim to stereotyped images of different economic, ethnic, or gender groups? It must be remembered that often the differences found within groups are often as strong as those that are found between groups. Ethnic differences, however, of both persons of color and of European descent, are fast becoming the linchpin that will be holding our country together. This is true now, but especially in the future, a future in which the majority of persons and workers in our country will be women and from groups of color.

The implications of these changing differences will have profound effects on the family policies that will address the children and families within our society. As theories are formulated, academic researchers will need to be brought out of the isolation of the ivory towers to collaborate with families within communities. There is need to go beyond the "short fix" reality of programs to more lasting solutions of the problems that blight the communities across this country. Together, academics, practitioners, funders of programs, and families themselves must be able to collaboratively design and implement policies and programs that will alleviate the mundane and acute stressors of their environments. The family policies that are developed will now need to incorporate these expanded rules of development.

The complexity of the developmental and contextual differences of individuals and families will provide the resources from which policies must be developed. This is especially apparent in the policies related to adolescents who become parents. Among all parents, the socialization goals for infant parenting are the development of healthy and secure young children. However, adolescent parents are at greater risk, developmentally and financially, of not meeting these goals. These adolescents require supportive social contexts to meet the challenges of too-early parenting. Social capital will facilitate the development of children to be able to offset the ravages that poverty may bring to their families.

The policies that are built into welfare systems will need to be more aware of the functional systems of these collaborative policy efforts. These multi-generational interventions will tend to promote family functioning and self-sufficiency. The abilities of families, their young, and their older members, to meet the socialization goals of the maintenance of families in stable positions, is the overall objective of a developmental systems perspective. Lerner, Sparks, and McCubbin have successfully articulated the impact of family diversity upon family policies. They are to be congratulated for the magnificent effort that they have made in pulling all of these varied perspectives together. All of these perspectives will be needed to go on to develop successful family policies and programs that will enhance the functioning of families.

REFERENCES

Bronfenbrenner, U. (1979). *The ecology of human development.* Cambridge, MA: Harvard University Press.
Elder, G. H., Jr., Modell, J., & Parke, R. D. (Eds.). (1993). *Children in time and place: Developmental and historical insights.* New York: Cambridge University Press.

PREFACE

The purpose of this book is to describe the dimensions of diversity that characterize the contemporary American family and, as well, to discuss the implications for public policies and associated intervention programs that may be linked to this diversity. Our view is that if the programs that are available to support families, and the rules or principles from which these programs are derived—that is, the policies pertinent to families—are to be maximally useful, they need to be developed to fit the characteristics of diversity of the families they are intended to help (Lerner, Sparks, & McCubbin, in press).

There is considerable theoretical and empirical work that underscores the importance of this book's purposes (e.g., Bronfenbrenner, 1974, 1979; Garbarino, 1992; Hahn, 1994; McAdoo, 1998; McLoyd, 1994; Philips & Bridgman, 1995; Pittman & Zeldin, 1994). This scholarship indicates that to adequately link family diversity and family policy we need to ask two questions: What sorts of families do we find in contemporary America? How are these families comparable to those that existed in prior decades?

These questions capture the two temporal (historical) perspectives that may be applied to the study of family diversity (Elder, 1974; Hernandez, 1993). Both are considered in this book in order to capture the plasticity of structure that characterizes the family and make inferences about the potential range of structural variation that might exist.

Accordingly, our book begins with a discussion of the historical and contemporary context of the American family—of the point-in-time and cross-time components of family life (Hernandez, 1993). This opening discussion leads to an analysis of perhaps the key contemporary challenge facing scholars and policy makers interested in understanding the import of family diversity for family policy: child poverty (Huston, 1991; McLoyd, 1994; Philips & Bridgman, 1995). We argue that this topic—involving non-random representations of racial and ethnic minorities among the poor children and families of our nation (Huston, 1991)—may be usefully studied within the context of a theoretical model that systematically links the development of individually different individuals to the variation that exists in their physical and social ecology (e.g., Bronfenbrenner, 1979). The instance of such a developmental systems model that we employ—developmental contextualism (Lerner, 1998)—is the topic of a subsequent chapter in which we describe how developmental contextualism, and developmental systems theory more broadly, serves as a frame for a presentation of the substantive issues pertinent to family structure and function that may be treated by a theoretically-informed focus on diversity.

To illustrate the usefulness of our approach to understanding the association between family diversity and family policy, we review data pertinent to three sample cases. First, we discuss the contemporary challenges faced by parents charged with rearing adolescents and, as well, the familial and societal issues that arise when those adolescents who are being reared are themselves parents (e.g., Lerner & Galambos, 1998). Second, we discuss current policy issues that arise from welfare debates in the United States and from the recently-enacted welfare reform legislation (e.g., Philips & Bridgman, 1995), indicating the importance of a focus on diversity in clarifying the controversies that have arisen with regard to specifying the rationale for, and implications for children of, welfare reform. Third, we discuss the importance for our nation of developing a national youth policy (we are the only Western nation without such a policy) and why such a development in policy may be formulated in relation to an understanding of the diversity of youth and their families (Hahn, 1994; Pittman & Zeldin, 1994).

We extract from the presentation of these three sample cases implications for the design, delivery, and evaluation of diversity-sensitive policies and programs for families and youth (Lerner, 1995). These implications are the focus of Chapter 8. This final chapter includes also a brief recapitulation of our key points in the volume, coupled with a vision of how to link scholars, policy makers, and community members in multi-professional and multi-institutional collaborations promoting the positive development of American families and youth. We describe some examples of models of such collaboration and conclude with some suggested action items that collaborators might pursue to begin to enact the vision on a more general basis than currently exists.

AUDIENCE

We intend this volume to be relevant to scholars of the family, of human development (and particularly of child and adolescent development), and of public policy. In addition, we hope that the volume will be attractive to policy makers—in government, industry/business, and public and private social service organizations (e.g., state family assistance agencies, and non-profit and for-profit providers of mental health services). In fact, we believe that those practitioners who, on a daily basis, have to address issues raised by working with diverse families within a policy context not sufficiently sensitive to diversity will find reason to be interested in this book.

We hope that our book will describe for these audiences the ways in which the issues raised by family diversity impact the current public policy system and, in turn, will suggest reasons for, and potential directions of, revisions of this system. Our intent is to offer an understanding of—and a vision for the further development of diversity-sensitive public policies for—our nation's diverse families and youth. We hope that this book will, therefore, clarify our present and provide a productive guide for our future.

ACKNOWLEDGMENTS

Several people were instrumental in the development of this book. The impetus for this book arose from an invitation we received to contribute to the *Handbook of Family Diversity*, edited by David Demo, Mark Fine, and Katherine Allen (Oxford University Press, in press). The chapter we prepared in response to this invitation provided a basis for the material we have developed for this volume. We are grateful to Drs. Demo, Fine, and Allen for their sage editorial feedback regarding our chapter in their volume and for the opportunity their invitation provided for us to think more broadly about the issues we introduced in the chapter for their volume. We are grateful as well to the several colleagues whose feedback about the drafts of all or portions of this volume sharpened our presentation and our thinking. In particular, we would like to thank Karen Bogenschneider and Harriette Pipes McAdoo for the excellent scholarship they have generated pertinent to the foci of this book and for their gracious collegiality in their writing such generous forewords to the volume. We are also grateful to Sofia T. Romero, editor at the Boston College Center for Child, Family, and Community Partnerships, for her expert and sage editing of this volume. Her skill, acumen, and guidance are deeply appreciated.

Finally, we express our gratitude to our respective families. Their support and devotion throughout the preparation of this book was an indispensable contribution for its completion. We dedicate this book to them.

REFERENCES

Bronfenbrenner, U. (1974). Developmental research, public policy, and the ecology of childhood. *Child Development, 45*, 1-5.

Bronfenbrenner, U. (1979). *The ecology of human development.* Cambridge, MA: Harvard University Press.

Elder, G. H., Jr. (1974). *Children of the Great Depression: Social change in life experiences.* Chicago: University of Chicago Press.

Garbarino, J. (1992). *Children and families in the social environment* (2nd ed.). New York: Aldine de Gruyter.

Hahn, A. B. (1994). Towards a national youth development policy for young African-American males: The choices policymakers face. In R. B. Mincy (Ed.), *Nurturing young black males: Challenges to agencies, programs, and social policy* (pp. 165-186). Washington, DC: The Urban Institute Press.

Hernandez, D. J. (1993). *America's children: Resources from family, government, and the economy.* New York: Russell Sage Foundation.

Huston, A. C. (Ed.). (1991). *Children in poverty: Child development and public policy.* Cambridge: Cambridge University Press.

Lerner, R. M. (1995). *America's youth in crisis: Challenges and options for programs and policies.* Thousand Oaks, CA: Sage.

Lerner, R. M. (1998). Theories of human development: Contemporary perspectives. In W. Damon (Series Ed.) & R. M. Lerner (Vol. Ed.), *Handbook of child psychology: Vol. 1 Theoretical models of human development* (5th ed., pp. 1-24). New York: Wiley.

Lerner, R. M., & Galambos, N. L. (1998). Adolescent development: Challenges and opportunities for research, programs, and policies. In J. T. Spence (Ed.), *Annual Review of Psychology* (Vol. 49, pp. 413-446). Palo Alto, CA: Annual Reviews.

Lerner, R. M., Sparks, E., & McCubbin, L. (In press). Family diversity and family policy. In D. Demo, K. Allen, & M. Fine (Eds.), *Handbook of family diversity.* New York: Oxford University Press.

McAdoo, H. (1998). African American families: Strength and realities. In H. McCubbin, E. Thompson, & J. Futrell, (Eds.), *Resiliency in ethnic minority families: African American families* (pp. 17-30). Thousand Oaks, CA: Sage.

McLoyd, V. C. (1994). Research in the service of poor and ethnic/racial minority children: A moral imperative. *Family and Consumer Sciences Research Journal, 23*, 56-66.

Phillips, D. A., & Bridgman, A. (Eds.). (1995). *New findings on children, families, and economic self-sufficiency: summary of a research briefing.* Washington, D.C.: National Academy Press.

Pittman, K. J., & Zeldin, S. (1994). From deterrence to development: Shifting the focus of youth programs for African-American males. In R. B. Mincy (Ed.), *Nurturing young black males: Challenges to agencies, programs, and social policy* (pp. 45-55). Washington, DC: The Urban Institute Press.

1 THE FAMILY: HISTORICAL AND CONTEMPORARY PERSPECTIVES

The lives and personal experiences of the authors reflect the key focus of this book: the relation between family diversity and family policy. Each of the three authors of this book are of different racial backgrounds and of different religions. Both genders are represented in the authorship team, and across the team there exist age differences of more than a generation. In turn, while all authors have immediate and extended families that span multiple generations, our locations in these generational groups vary. For instance, one author is a member of the youngest generation in her family constellation whereas another author is the parent of several teenagers and, at the same time, contributes to the support of an aged mother. Add to this diversity the fact that across their respective lives the authors have had experiences with their immediate and extended families that pertained to both normative life events such as births, deaths, marriages and divorces, and to non-normative life events such as unexpected illnesses, changes in family structure, financial calamities, and severe accidents.

Together, these lifetimes of personal and experiential diversity have resulted in the authors seeking and receiving emotional, physical, and even financial support or assistance from immediate and extended family members, from neighbors and friends, and from community institutions (e.g., from religious institutions, civic societies, or governmental bodies). At times, this support was just what was needed to match the particular circumstances faced by one of us. At other times, however, the programs that were available to help us cope with life events did not match the individuality of our situation. We have learned, then, both through our scholarship and through our personal lives, that if the programs that are available to support families, and the rules or principles from which these programs are derived, that is, the policies pertinent to families, are to be maximally useful, they need to be developed to fit the characteristics of diversity of the families they are intended to help.

A FOCUS ON FAMILIES AND CHILDREN

We believe that the key function of the family—historically, and even evolutionarily (Lerner, 1984; Lerner & Spanier, 1978, 1980)—is to represent in institutional context that is best able to insure the survival and socialization of children. The family is the institution charged with children to be committed to the maintenance and perpetuation of the cultural context within which they develop. Through such rearing, the family is the key institution contributing to the maintenance and perpetuation of society (Lerner, 1984; Lerner & Spanier, 1978, 1980).

Accordingly, society must develop principles or strategies—policies, if you will—that enable all families to produce children capable of, and committed to, contributing to self and society in a positive and integrated way. In other words, in the superordinate sense of enabling civil society to be maintained and perpetuated, all families with children—no matter what their particular structure may be (e.g., families wherein two biological parents rear children; families wherein step parents are involved in child rearing; families with adopted children; or single-parent families)—have the responsibility of socializing the next generation in ways that allow children to become productive and committed members of society. Any society, then, needs to develop rules about families—family policies—that enable such contributions to be made by the diverse families that exist within it.

Clearly, then, the approach we take to the family is one that emphasizes its contributions to promoting positive, healthy child development. We focus on the family as a social institution that functions to maintain and perpetuate society through the rearing of children. Certainly, it is possible to have a family without children; that is, we would not deny that two adults married or permanently committed to each other can maintain with legitimacy that they are a family. Indeed, such structures are part of what we would include in any description of the full range of diverse contemporary families. However, our interest in this book is to focus on families with children and how, through developing policies that better serve the diversity that exists among such families, we can strengthen the ability of families to promote positive child development.

FAMILY DIVERSITY AND FAMILY POLICY: KEY QUESTIONS

To adequately link family diversity and family policy in our nation we need to ask two questions: What sorts of families do we find in contemporary America? How are these families comparable to those that existed in prior decades?

These questions capture the two temporal perspectives that may be applied to the study of family diversity. The former question is predicated on a point-in-time, or cross-sectional, perspective. The latter question is derived from an interest in cross-time, longitudinal analysis. Both temporal perspectives are needed to appreciate the plasticity of structure that characterizes the family and to make inferences about the potential range of structural variation that might exist. The presence of potential variation—not only in structure but as well in function—is vital if policies are to be realistic guides for actions that can effect desired changes (Lerner, 1984).

Public policies represent standards, or rules, for the conduct of individuals, organizations, and institutions. The policies that we formulate and follow structure our actions and enunciate to others how they may expect us to function with regard to the substantive issues to which our policies pertain. Moreover, our policies reflect what we value, what we believe, and what we think is in our best interests; they indicate the things in which we are invested and about which we care. Public policies aimed at enhancing the family are, implicitly, temporal initiatives. They are social actions designed to change family structure or function from a "status" at one point in time to a "status" at another point in time. Inherently, then, policies also have to be seen in the context of the same two temporal parameters within which the study of family diversity is embedded. The cross-sectional and longitudinal diversity of family structures may provide practical boundaries framing the changes that policies seek to create. In turn, the temporal parameters of family diversity give some empirical justification that there is plasticity in family structure (and, it may be analogously argued, in family function) sufficient to enable public policies to create theoretically inferred, new forms of the family.

In short, then, temporality is a key parameter of both family diversity and family policy. It is useful, then, to discuss the point-in-time and cross-time components of family.

The first author of this book grew up at a time when the stereotypic White American family was an intact nuclear one, with two biological parents and two or three children (named either David and Ricky, or Bud, Kitten, and Princess, respectively). Yet, today, only one in five married couples with children fits this still popular stereotype of living in what has been termed the "Ozzie and Harriet" family, i.e., the intact, never-divorced, two-parent-two-child family (Ahlburg & De Vita, 1992; Hernandez, 1993). For African American and Latino children, there are even fewer children who are living in two-parent families where the father is the bread-winner and the mother is a homemaker. Indeed, as shown in Table 1.1, at any one time children and parents may live in several quite different family contexts (see Allison, 1993; Lerner, Castellino, Terry, Villarruel, & McKinney, 1995).

This diversity of family structures or, at the least, of contexts serving the socialization functions of families (Lerner & Spanier, 1978, 1980), requires a definition of family broader than one pointing to an intact nuclear family wherein parents raise their biological children. As such, we see a family as not merely a household. Rather, it is an institution wherein individuals, related through biology or enduring social commitments, and representing similar or different generations and/or genders, engage in roles involving mutual socialization, nurturance, and emotional exchange. The number of children living in many of the types of family contexts shown in Table 1.1 has increased dramatically in recent years. As an example consider the category of foster care homes. Between 1987 and 1991, the number of children in foster care increased by more than 50%, from 300,000 to 460,000 (Carnegie Corporation of New York, 1994). Infants less than 12 months old are among the age groups of children most likely to be placed in such care (Carnegie Corporation of New York, 1994). As with many of the other statistics that refer to children living in poverty and non-traditional family arrangements, the percentage of children of color is disproportionately higher than for European Americans. Virtually all of the zip code areas having the highest placement rates also have the lowest level of family incomes, and the children are predominantly

Table 1.1
Some of the contemporary "family" contexts of children and youth

>Intact nuclear (biological)
>Single parent (biological)
>Intact nuclear (adoptive)
>Single parent (adoptive)
>Intact (blended)
>>(Heterosexual; Gay; Lesbian)
>
>Single parent (step)
>Intergenerational
>Extended, without parent
>>(e.g., child-aunt)
>
>*In loco parentis* families/institutions
>>Foster care homes
>>Group homes
>>Psychiatric hospitals
>>Residential treatment facilities
>>Juvenile detention facilities
>
>Runaways
>Street children/youth
>>(e.g., Adolescent prostitutes)
>
>Homeless children

Source: Lerner, Castellino, et al., 1995

from ethnic minority groups (Wulczyn, 1994).

In addition, the cross-sectional location of people in one of the family contexts noted in Table 1.1 is complicated by the fact that such settings may change longitudinally over the course of the lives of children and parents, and thus across generations (i.e., across history). This observation raises the need for a historically-embedded "developmental demographics" of child-parent relations (Allison, 1993), a point underscored by the research of Featherman, Spenner, and Tsunematsu (1988) and, more recently, of Hernandez (1993). For instance, Featherman, et al. demonstrate that even with a contextual variable as seemingly general (and presumably somewhat stable) as social class, only approximately 46% of American children remain at age 6 years in the social class within which they were born. Indeed, about 22% of all children born in the United States change from their initial social class during their first year of life. Moreover, during the first six years of life about 54% of American children have lived in two or more social classes (Featherman et al., 1988). Given the fact that social class structures the large majority of the resources and cultural values influencing families, these magnitudes of change underscore the need to appraise the diversity of child-family relations longitudinally (historically) as well as cross-sectionally.

This viewpoint is brought to the fore by the scholarship of Hernandez (1993). Using census and survey data, Hernandez (1993) describes several quite profound changes that have characterized the life courses of America's children and their families over the last 50 to 150 years. Using the scholarship of Hernandez as a frame, we may discuss the history and current features of the American family and the potential impacts of these changes on the children of our nation.

HISTORICAL AND CONTEMPORARY VARIATION IN THE FAMILY: THE SCHOLARSHIP OF HERNANDEZ

Hernandez (1993) argues that a person's life trajectory is constituted by, and differentiated from, those of others on the basis of, the specific order, duration, and timing of the particular events and resources experienced in life, and by the number, characteristics, and activities of the family members with whom the person lives. Using this viewpoint as a frame, Hernandez describes what he labels as eight *revolutions* in the lives of America's children across this century.

The Disappearance of the Two-Parent Farm Family and the Growth of the One-Parent Family

Hernandez (1993) notes that between the late eighteenth century to almost the end of the nineteenth century the majority of American children lived in two-parent farm families during their first 17 years. These numbers differed for African American and other children of color since many lived in extreme poverty and in families that were negatively affected by economic hardships. At the beginning of the twentieth century, about 40% of all children in this age range still lived in such family settings, with slightly more than an additional 40% living in nonfarm, two-parent families with the father as the "breadwinner" and the mother as the homemaker. The remaining children in this age range at the beginning of this century (slightly more than 10%) lived either in dual-earner nonfarm, or one parent, families or in no-parent situations. A larger percentage of African American children are reflected in this 10%, as the normative family arrangement within the African American community at that time was for both parents to be wage-earners, and there were many mother-only families.

By 1950, only about 15% of American children lived, during their first 17 years of life, in two-parent farm families, whereas almost 60% of American children in this age range lived in intact nonfarm families wherein the father was the breadwinner and the mother was the homemaker. Dual-earner nonfarm, or one parent, families were the settings wherein most of the remaining American children within this age range lived. As in the earlier periods in history, the actual percentages within the African American and other communities of color differed, with a greater percentage of the population in either dual-earner nonfarm families or single-parent households.

In 1990, however, fewer than 5% of America's children lived, during the first 17 years of their lives, in two-parent farm families. Moreover, fewer than 30% of children in this age range lived in intact nonfarm families wherein the father was the breadwinner and the mother was the homemaker. Rather, about 70% of all American children in this age range lived either in dual-earner nonfarm families or in one-parent families. Indeed, approximately 25% lived in one-parent families. When looking at the percentage of non-European American children living in dual-earner nonfarm families or in one-parent families, these numbers are significantly increased, with approximately 38.2% of African American and 34.2% of Puerto Rican children living in mother-only households in 1980.

In this regard, Hamburg (1992, p. 33) observes that:

> It is startling to realize that today most American children spend part of their childhood in a single-parent family. By age sixteen, close to half the children of married parents will see their parents divorce. Usually the child remains with the mother. For nearly half of these children, it will be five years or more before their mothers remarry. Close to half of all white children whose parents remarry will see the second marriage dissolve during their adolescence. Black women not only marry less often and experience more marital disruption, but also remarry more slowly and less often than white women. America exhibits a revolving-door pattern in marriage that is certainly stressful for developing children and adolescents.

Furthermore, the increase in one-parent families was coupled with a decrease across this century in the presence of a grandparent in the home. By 1990, about 80% of children in one-parent families did not live with a grandparent (U.S. Department of Commerce, 1993). Thus, the parenting resources accrued from having two adults in the home are generally absent in contemporary American one-parent families since in the majority of such families there is no grandparent present to replace the resources represented by the absent parent.

The Decrease in the Number of Siblings in the Family

In 1890, 46% of America's children lived in families wherein they had eight or more siblings. An additional 30% lived in families wherein they had between five and seven siblings, and 16% lived in families where they had either three or four siblings. Only 7% of America's children lived in families having either one or two siblings (Hernandez, 1993).

By 1940, however, families wherein a child had eight or more siblings accounted for only 10% of America's families. In turn, the percentages of American families wherein a child had either between five and seven siblings, three or four siblings, or only one or two siblings were 21%, 38%, and 30%, respectively (Hernandez, 1993).

In 1990, however, only one percent of America's children lived in families wherein they had eight or more siblings. In addition, only 5% of America's children lived in families with five to seven siblings, and about an additional 38% lived in

Family Diversity and Family Policy

families wherein they had either three or four siblings. In turn, about 57% lived in families with either one or two siblings (Hernandez, 1993).

This change in the number of siblings in the home has been coupled with a corresponding decrease in the average size of households in America. Indeed, Hamburg (1992) notes that the size of the average American household has diminished to its smallest level ever. Moreover he notes that:

> One-quarter of the nation's households consist of people living alone. This is twenty-three million individuals. The change has come rapidly. The number of people living alone more than doubled between 1970 and 1990—yet another indication of the dramatic transformation of American families taking place in recent decades. While this finding has positive as well as negative implications, it certainly highlights a major challenge to the adequacy of social supports under the transforming conditions of contemporary life. (Hamburg, 1992, pp. 12-13)

The Increase in Parents' Education

Hernandez (1993) reports that in the 1920s about 60% of the children in America had fathers with at least eight years of schooling, whereas about 15% of America's children had fathers with at least four years of high school education. The corresponding rates for mothers were a few percentage points higher than those for fathers.

In the 1950s, parental educational attainment had markedly increased. Approximately 90% of all mothers, and about 87% of all fathers, had eight or more years of schooling. In turn, 60% of mothers, and about 55% of fathers, had at least four years of high school (Hernandez, 1993).

To the end of the 1980s these trends of increasing levels of parental education continued. By that time about 96% of all mothers and fathers had eight or more years of schooling. Moreover, about 80% of all mothers and about 85% of all fathers had at least four years of high school (Hernandez, 1993). These statistics reflect trends for all children, regardless of race.

However, when looking specifically at ethnic-minority families, the trends are somewhat different. Despite a substantial narrowing of the racial gap in parents' education, African American children continue to be at a disadvantage and lag substantially behind European American children in their chances of having parents who have completed at least four years of high school or college. For Latino children, by the 1970s cohort, old-family Latino children (of any race) and non-Hispanic Blacks were about equal in their chances of being educationally disadvantaged by family origins, and first-generation Latino children (of any race) were somewhat more disadvantaged. Latino children (of any race) born of parents in the United States by 1988 may continue to be fairly similar to non-Hispanic Blacks in their chances of being educationally disadvantaged by family origins (Hernandez, 1993).

The Growth of Mothers in the Labor Force

As documented by Hernandez (1993) and by J. Lerner (1994), the percentage of children with mothers in the labor force has increased dramatically across the last half century. Indeed, in 1940 only 10% of America's children had mothers in the labor force. In 1950, this percentage had only grown to 16%. However, in 1960 more than one quarter (26%) of America's children had "working mothers," and by 1970 this proportion had grown to greater than one third (36%). In turn, in 1980 49% of America's children had mothers in the labor force, and by 1990 this figure had grown to 59% (Hernandez, 1993). Similarly, while in 1950 14% of women in the United States with children under six years of age were in the labor force, in 1990 the corresponding rate was 58% (Morelli & Verhoef, in press).

Within the African American community, these numbers have been higher since the 1920s, when Black women entered the labor force in large numbers in order to help support their families. In 1980, statistics indicate that 53.1% of all African American families were in the labor force and, by 1995, this number had increased to 59.5%. The number of African American women with children who are in the labor force and who are living with a spouse are even higher, with 76.3% of African American mothers with children under three years of age and 77.3% with children under six years being in the labor force.

Moreover, as noted by Hamburg (1992) and J. Lerner (1994), this increase in maternal employment impacts on child and adolescent development is as yet incompletely understood or documented ways. For example, Hamburg (1992, pp. 10-11) notes that:

> As women have opened up unprecedented opportunities for themselves and are making an enormous contribution to the well-being of the economy and the society, they have less time for their children. By and large, fathers and grandparents simply are not compensating for this historical shift.
>
> So families are living in a time of flux. It is a time of magnificent opportunities and of insidious stress. Just as the economic functions of the family moved out of the home early in the Industrial Revolution, so child-care functions, too, are now moving outside the home to a large extent. The child's development is less and less under parents' and grandparents' direct supervision and increasingly placed in the hands of strangers and near-strangers. In the main, this transformation was unforeseen and unplanned, and it is still poorly understood.

One of the unplanned features of this transformation is that, in 1994, more than five million American children under three years of age were in the care of other adults when their parent or parents were at work. As noted by the Carnegie Corporation of New York (1994), much of the care received by these young children is of poor quality.

Changes in Fathers' Full-Time Employment

The marked growth in maternal employment since 1940 has been coupled with the fact that, between the 1940s and the 1980s, many of America's children lived with fathers who were not employed full-time year-round (Hernandez, 1993). In 1940, 40% of America's children lived with fathers who did not have full-time employment all year. In 1950, this rate fell to 32% and, by 1980, it fell still further to 24%.

However, between 1950 and 1980, the 8% decrease in children living with fathers who did not have full-time employment was offset by an 8% increase in children who did not have a father in the home (Hernandez, 1993). Given the percentage of American children that lived in such father-absent homes during this period, Hernandez (1993) notes that, from the 1950s to the 1980s, only about 60% of America's children lived with fathers who worked full-time all of the year.

The Growth of Single-Parent, Female Head-of-Household Families

During the last half century there has been a dramatic increase in the percentage of American children living with only their mothers (Hernandez, 1993). In 1940, 1950, and 1960, the proportion of children living in single-parent, female head-of-household families remained relatively steady, with 6.7%, 6.4%, and 7.7%, respectively, of children living in such households. However, between 1960 and 1990, the percentage of children living in such families almost tripled. In 1970, the percentage was 11.8%, in 1980 it was 16.2%, and in 1990 it was 20% (Hernandez, 1993). These percentages are higher within non-European American families.

In addition to out-of-wedlock births, a major reason for the growth of single-parent, female head-of-household families is the rising divorce rate in America. As noted by the Carnegie Corporation of New York (1994), in 1906, less than 1% of children per year experienced the divorce of their parents. However, by 1993, almost 50% of all children could expect to experience the divorce of their parents; for non-European American children, these figures are even higher. On the average European American children live five years in a single parent family; for African American children, this period tends to be longer.

The Disappearance of the "Ozzie and Harriet" Family (i.e., the Intact, Never Divorced, Two Parent-Two Child Family)

Over the course of the twentieth century, America has experienced a disappearance of the stereotypically predominant intact, two-parent family, wherein the father is the breadwinner, the mother is the homemaker, and two to three children either spend their lives in socioeconomic and personal security or are faced with problems that require only about 30 minutes (the time of the typical American television situation comedy) to resolve. Hernandez (1993) demonstrates that not only are such stereotypic family milieus largely absent in America but, since the 1940s, a decreasing minority of children have been born into such families.

Hamburg (1992) notes that until the beginning of the 1960s, most of the people in the United States believed that much of this stereotype was, in fact, true. Specifically, Hamburg (1992, p. 32) indicates that Americans believed that:

1. A family consists of a husband and wife living together with their children.
2. The father is the head of the family and should earn the family's income and give his name to his wife and children.
3. The mother's main tasks are to support and facilitate the work of her husband, guide her children's development, look after the home, and set a moral tone for the family.
4. Marriage is an enduring obligation for better and worse; the husband and wife have the joint task of coping with stresses, including those of the child's development; and sexual activity, especially by women, should be kept within the marriage.
5. Parents have an overriding responsibility for the well-being of their children during their early years; until they enter school, the parents have almost sole responsibility, and even later must be the primary guardians of their children's education and discipline.

While Hamburg (1992) stresses that Americans were aware that these beliefs were not necessarily readily actualized, the beliefs nevertheless represented ideals against which actual families were compared.

In 1940, 1950, 1960, and 1970, the percentage of children born into "Ozzie and Harriet" type European American families was 40.8%, 44.5%, 43.1%, and 37.3%, respectively. However, by 1980, this percentage fell to 27.4% (Hernandez, 1993). Moreover, few Americans spend their entire childhood and adolescent years in such family settings. Indeed, in 1920, only 31% of children and youth lived their first 17 years in these types of families. This percentage fell to 16.3% by 1960, and estimates for succeeding decades have fallen to less than 10% (Hernandez, 1993)

The Growth of Marriage by Cohabitation

Two new family patterns that are emerging also increase the diversity of the family structure in contemporary American society: cohabitation and stepparent families (Bumpass & Sweet, 1989). Families formed by cohabitation, i.e., by living together without marriage, have increased while marriage rates have fallen (Bumpass & Sweet, 1989). Marriages preceded by cohabitation can be short-lived and are more likely to end in a divorce (Bumpass, Raley, & Sweet, 1994).

According to Bumpass, Raley, and Sweet (1994), cohabitation for men has increased from 8% in 1940 to 33% in 1964. Marriages for men decreased from 68% in 1949 to 38% in 1964. For women, cohabitation increased from 3% in 1940 to

37% in 1964. Marriages for women decreased from 82% in 1949 to 61% in 1964. Among African American families estimates are that 29% of families are formed through cohabitation; among European Americans, 20% of families are formed through cohabitation; and for Mexican Americans, 21% of families are formed through cohabitation (Bumpass, Raley, & Sweet, 1994). Of these families, only one in ten are still cohabiting after 10 years.

Thus, in the context of the disappearance of the Ozzie and Harriet family and of current rates of divorce and of non-marital childbearing, cohabitation is a factor that is reshaping the range of diversity of family structures in America. Indeed, one fourth of unwed mothers are cohabiting with the child's father at the time of birth (Bumpass, Raley, & Sweet, 1994).

The substitution of cohabitation for marriage and remarriage means that many children will gain a stepparent by a parent's cohabitation rather than through parental marriage. One third of women are likely to live in a family involving arrangements of stepparenting caused by marriage/remarriage and one fourth of children will have lived in a family with stepparents (Bumpass, Raley, & Sweet, 1994). However, when cohabiting is included in the definition of a stepparenting family, 40% of women and 30% of all children spend time in such a family unit. A higher proportion of African American mothers (50%) and African American children (40%) will live in this type of stepfamily, despite the lower rates of marriage and remarriage among African Americans. Indeed, one third of the children entering stepfamilies do so after birth to an unwed mother rather than after a divorce or separation, and about two thirds enter through cohabitation (Bumpass, Raley, & Sweet, 1994). Two thirds of African American families and 55% of European American families create stepparent families by cohabitation (Bumpass, Raley, & Sweet, 1994).

About 25% of cohabiting stepfamilies marry within one year and 50% marry within five years (Bumpass, Raley, & Sweet, 1994). Nearly one half (40%) of the children in stepfamilies created by cohabitation experience family disruption in five years. However, 60% of such families are still intact after five years (Bumpass, Raley, & Sweet, 1994). When compared with stepfamilies created by marriage over a 10 year period, there is no difference between stepfamilies formed by cohabitation versus stepfamilies created by marriages. Both types of families have a 50% rate of disruption. In turn, 60% of stepfamily units are intact after seven years whether they are begun by cohabitation or by marriage.

The Reappearance of Wide-Spread Child Poverty

A final revolution described by Hernandez (1993) pertains to the changing distribution of children across relative income levels and, as such, to a growth of child poverty, especially during the 1980s. After the Great Depression the relative poverty rate among children dropped from 38% in 1939 to 27% in 1949 (Hernandez, 1993). During the 1950s, this rate dropped to 24% and, by 1969, the rate was 23% (Hernandez, 1993).

However, between 1969 and 1988, this trend of decreasing relative poverty among children reversed and, by 1988, relative poverty among children had grown by 4% (Hernandez, 1993). In other words, during the 1980s, the percentage of children living in poor families returned to the comparatively high level seen about 40 years earlier, in 1949 (Hernandez, 1993). Through 1997, this level of poverty did not abate (The Annie E. Casey Foundation, 1997). Moreover, the percentage of children living in "middle-class comfort" decreased between 1969 and 1988 from 43% to 37% (Hernandez, 1993).

Although most children in poverty are European American, a disproportionate number of children in poverty are African American and Latino. The trends in poverty rates for these non-European American groups has tended to follow a similar pattern through the years (Child Welfare League, 1993).

From Historical Changes to Contemporary Issues Associated with Child and Family Poverty

In sum, Hernandez (1993) embeds the child-parent relation within an historically changing matrix of variables involving family structure and function and other key institutions of society (e.g., the educational system and the economy). The import of Hernandez's scholarship for the present discussion is that the American family is a product of multidimensional historical changes in the contexts of family life. As such, historical variation provides both a basis for the diversity of the family that exists at any point in time and suggests the parameters of changes that may influence the future course of these diverse relations. Indeed, the importance of focusing on an historically embedded analysis of diversity in the American family is further underscored by an appraisal of the contemporary differences in family-child relations that exist across socioeconomic settings (i. e., among the poor and non-poor), and in relation to different racial/ethnic groups.

The diversity that exists in contemporary American families is dramatically seen when we examine the effects of poverty on children. McAdoo (1998a) sees poverty as the greatest challenge to resiliency for African American families. It is very appropriate, then, to turn to a discussion of child poverty in America, because of the "rotten outcomes" (Schorr, 1988) linked to poverty in regard to family life and child development.

2 CHILD POVERTY WITHIN THE ECOLOGY OF AMERICA'S FAMILIES

By the end of the 1980s, approximately 20% of America's children were poor, an increase across the decade of 17% in the national rate of child poverty. Moreover, Phillips and Bridgman (1995, p. 1) note that in 1993 "poverty among American children reached its highest level in 30 years." Indeed, 22.7% (or 15.7 million) of America's children were poor in 1993 (Bureau of the Census, 1994). Moreover, as noted in Chapter 1, there was no improvement in the rate of child poverty in America during the latter years of the twentieth century.

CONTEMPORARY INCIDENCE OF CHILD POVERTY

As summarized by the Annie E. Casey Foundation in the *Kids Count Data Book* (1997, pp. 16-17):

> The Percent of Children in Poverty is perhaps the most global and widely used indicator of child well-being. This is due, in part, to the fact that poverty is closely linked to a number of undesirable outcomes in areas such as health, education, emotional well-being, and delinquency. The data shown here are based on the government's official poverty measure ($15, 569 for a family of four in 1995).
>
> Between 1985 and 1994, there was no change in the poverty rate of children (21 percent), but this masks countervailing trends during this period. National data show that the poverty rate among related children (under age 18) declined from 1985 to 1989, increased from 19.0 percent to 22.0 percent in 1993, before inching downward to 21.2 percent in 1994 and 20.2 percent in 1995.
>
> Children born to parents who have not graduated from high school have a strong likelihood of growing up in poverty. In 1995 the poverty rate for children living with parents who dropped out of high school was 57 percent, compared to 4 percent for children who have at least one parent who obtained a college degree.

Despite the enormous wealth in the United States, our child poverty rate is among the highest in the developed world. One study which examined child poverty rates in 17 developed countries indicates that the child poverty rate in the United States is 50 percent higher than the next highest rate. The gap in the child poverty rate between the United States and other developed countries is a product of differences in private sector income, but the gap is greatly accentuated by enormous differences in the role government plays in alleviating child poverty. This lack of investment in our children will put us at a competitive disadvantage in the international marketplace of the 21st century.

In 1994 there were 10 states and the District of Columbia where a quarter or more of all children were poor. In 1994 the child poverty rate ranged from a low of 9 percent in New Hampshire to a high of 37 percent in the District of Columbia.

Confirming the findings reported in the 1997 *Kids Count Data Book* that there is substantial variation across states in youth poverty, the National Center for Children in Poverty (1998) reported that seven states and the District of Columbia have young child poverty rates significantly higher than the national average and 15 states have rates that are significantly lower. Table 2.1 presents these data.

In addition, other data summarized in Table 2.1 indicate that 10 states have experienced significant changes in the young child poverty rates since the period from 1979 to 1983. Eight states have seen their rates increase but only two states have seen their rates decrease. In fact, our nation's three largest states—California, New York, and Texas—alone accounted for more than 50% of the increase of 1.5 million children in poverty in the period from 1978/1983 to 1992/1996 (National Center for Children in Poverty, 1998). Moreover, across all states, the National Center for Children in Poverty found that three demographic factors accounted for a substantial proportion of the changes in rates of child poverty. These demographic factors are:

> the proportions of young children with: (1) single mothers (family structure), (2) mothers who completed high school (parental education), and (3) at least one parent employed full-time (parental employment). (National Center for Children in Poverty, 1998, p. 2)

The latter two variables are inversely related to poverty rates, whereas the first variable is positively related to poverty rate.

Although showing geographic variation, data from both the Annie E. Casey Foundation (1997) and the National Center for Children in Poverty (1998) indicate that poverty is a persistent and pervasive issue facing our nation. However, as noted in Chapter 1, poverty is not equally or randomly distributed among the diverse citizens of America. Poverty exists with different probability among different racial/ethnic groups (Center for the Study of Social Policy, 1993). In 1989, 44% of

Family Diversity and Family Policy

Table 2.1
Change in the percentage and number of children under age six in poverty, by state, 1979-1983 to 1992-1996

	1979–1983		1992–1996		% Change in rate	Change in number
	Rate	Number	Rate	Number		
USA	22.04	4,420,791	24.67	5,877,075	12	1,456,284
Connecticut	14.75	30,440	23.96	67,250	62	36,810
Wyoming	12.50	6,075	19.38	7,710	55	1,635
Oklahoma	20.94	54,643	32.03	92,384	53	37,741
Montana	17.22	14,626	25.95	20,019	51	5,393
Arizona	19.76	49,025	28.89	124,350	46	75,325
West Virginia	27.65	48,739	39.99	47,962	45	-777
Louisiana	29.14	133,557	40.65	158,447	40	24,890
Kentucky	21.37	73,950	29.37	90,042	37	16,092
District of Columbia	33.09	13,791	44.17	23,424	33	9,632
Maryland	13.94	40,545	18.57	94,425	33	53,879
Texas	24.39	358,482	30.27	572,180	24	213,698
California	23.40	516,759	28.97	950,269	24	433,510
Missouri	19.38	81,911	23.95	102,202	24	20,291
New York	23.75	338,754	28.76	464,551	21	125,797
Minnesota	14.30	55,640	17.19	68,142	20	12,503
Ohio	19.55	188,078	23.06	223,470	18	35,392
New Mexico	28.82	39,598	33.99	58,049	18	18,450
North Carolina	20.90	94,869	24.59	144,267	18	49,398
Nevada	14.22	10,790	16.63	20,938	17	10,148
North Dakota	14.79	9,744	17.26	8,613	17	-1,131
Michigan	22.82	188,947	25.75	225,755	13	36,809
Maine	20.20	18,634	22.45	19,567	11	933
Massachusetts	14.99	66,137	16.65	84,557	11	18,420
Wisconsin	14.60	64,074	16.16	73,080	11	9,006
New Hampshire	10.85	7,761	11.85	12,236	9	4,475
Georgia	21.93	107,270	23.74	152,241	8	44,971
Kansas	18.84	41,567	20.23	50,245	7	8,678
Illinois	23.27	232,025	24.27	271,889	4	39,864
Indiana	20.60	107,121	21.47	118,010	4	10,889
Colorado	16.66	43,763	17.23	55,659	3	11,896
Iowa	16.64	41,564	17.09	45,228	3	3,664
Florida	26.35	199,106	26.55	313,231	1	114,125
Washington	18.31	69,858	18.44	89,168	1	19,310
Oregon	20.34	50,535	20.13	51,635	-1	1,101
Nebraska	19.42	29,290	18.71	29,478	-4	188
Tennessee	28.90	114,313	27.83	123,466	-4	9,153
Virginia	18.41	79,434	17.43	92,544	-5	13,110
Mississippi	38.01	87,044	35.49	86,319	-7	-726
South Carolina	25.90	88,330	23.99	74,702	-7	-13,628
Arkansas	30.04	60,633	27.02	59,990	-10	-643
Pennsylvania	20.60	179,593	18.38	179,569	-11	-23
Idaho	24.59	26,458	21.74	22,397	-12	-4,061
South Dakota	24.94	18,767	21.92	13,437	-12	-5,330
Rhode Island	24.47	16,862	20.39	15,266	-17	-1,596
Hawaii	22.03	20,490	18.35	19,015	-17	-1,475
Utah	14.14	32,778	11.36	26,338	-20	-6,440
Alabama	32.46	118,385	25.86	100,936	-20	-17,449
Alaska	18.01	9,452	13.78	8,749	-23	-703
Delaware	20.07	10,709	15.27	8,750	-24	-1,959
New Jersey	20.88	119,125	15.37	107,412	-26	-11,713
Vermont	21.91	10,754	13.31	7,521	-39	-3,233

* States in bold letters had significantly positive or significantly negative growth as indicated. Other states may have had similar changes but because of small sample sizes these changes are not considered statistically significant at a 90 percent confidence interval. Changes in poverty rates are rounded to the nearest whole number.

Source: Bennett & Li, 1998

African American children were poor, a rate four times greater than the corresponding one for European American children (Center for the Study of Social Policy, 1993). Among Latino children, the rate of child poverty in 1989 was 38%, and for these children the increase in child poverty across the 1980s was 25%, the greatest increase for any of America's racial/ethnic groups (Center for the Study of Social Policy, 1993). In terms of absolute numbers, data from the 1990 Census indicate that 5.9 million European American children lived in poverty, whereas the corresponding numbers of African Americans, Asian Americans, Native Americans, and Latinos were 3.7 million, 346,000, 260,000, and 2.4 million, respectively (Children's Defense Fund, 1992).

In short, as noted by Huston (1991), race is the most striking and disturbing distinction between children whose poverty is chronic and children for whom poverty is transitory. For instance, Duncan (1991) reports data from the Panel Study on Income Dynamics indicating that the average African American child in the study spent 5.5 years in poverty. In turn, the average non-African American child in the study spent only 0.9 years in poverty. Furthermore, as with race and ethnicity, poverty is not equally distributed across age groups. In 1989, about 20% of children younger than age 6 years were poor, and the corresponding rate of poverty for 6- to 17-year-olds was about 17%. In turn, the rates for Americans aged 18 to 64 years, or aged 65 years or older, were about 11% and 13%, respectively (Children's Defense Fund, 1992).

Across the 1980s, there was a 13% increase in the number of children living in single-parent families, a trend present in 44 states. Thus, from 1987 to 1991, 18.1%, 30% and 56.7% of European American, Latino, and African American children, respectively, lived in single-parent households (Center for the Study of Social Policy, 1992). Most of these single-parent households are female-headed, and the poverty rates in such households were, by the beginning of the 1990s, 29.8% for European American families, 50.6% for African American families, and 53% for Latino families (U.S. Department of Commerce, 1991). In turn, 34.2% of households of 25 of the largest Native American tribes in 1989 were single-parent families and of these, 27.2% were living in poverty. Since the income of female-headed, single-parent families is often three or more times lower than two-parent families, and is also lower than single-parent, male-headed families, the fact that increasing numbers of children live in these family structures means that the financial resources to support parenting are less likely to be available (Center for the Study of Social Policy, 1993).

As the poverty rates of America's children worsen, exceeding now all other major industrialized nations (Huston, 1991), the structure of the family is also changing in ways that have placed poor children and parents at greater risk to problems of family life and individual development (Hernandez, 1993). To illustrate, in 1990, 90.3% of children were living with their parents, 7.3% were living with other relatives, and 2.3% were living outside of the family (Center for the Study of Social Policy, 1992). However, only 41.9% of African American children, 67.7% of Latino children, and 78.5% of European American children between the ages of 10 and 14 lived with both their parents (Simons, Finlay, & Yang, 1991). In turn, between the ages of 15 and 17, only 41%, 63%, and 76% of

African American, Latino, and European American children, respectively, live in two-parent families (Simons, et al., 1991) According to Reddy (1993), only about half of all Native American families consist of traditional "two-parent biological" families.

INDIVIDUAL AND FAMILY PROBLEMS ASSOCIATED WITH POVERTY

These trends involving child poverty, and the family structure and parenting resources to which poor children have access, are associated with problems of family life and child development. For instance, there is substantial information suggesting that the influence on children of family economic adversity is likely to be strong and negative (e.g., see Huston, 1991).

To illustrate, according to data presented in the 1993 *Kids Count Data Book*, published by the Center for the Study of Social Policy, 1.7 million new American families were started in 1990 by the birth of a new baby. However, 45% of these new families were at major risk of experiencing problems such as having inadequate family resources (that is, of living below the poverty line) or witnessing negative developments for the child (e.g., poor school performance). These risks existed primarily because of the presence of at least one of three factors: (1) The mother had less than 12 years of schooling; (2) the mother was unmarried to the child's father; and (3) the mother was a teenager at the time of the birth of her first baby. Moreover, in 24% of new families, two of these risk factors were present, and in 11% all three risk factors were present.

That these risk factors are significant for family life and for child development can be illustrated further by reference to other 1993 *Kids Count Data Book* information linking these three risk factors to child poverty and to school achievement. Among all 7- to 12-year-old children living in America, there was a probability of .79 that the child would be poor if all three risk factors were present. Similarly, the probability of being in the lower half of one's school class was .58 if all these three factors were present. In turn, when any two of these risk factors were present the probability of being poor or of being in the bottom half of one's school class was .48 and .53, respective. The corresponding probabilities involving the presence of only one risk factor were .26 and .47, respectively. Moreover, when none of these risk factors were present the probability of 7- to 12-year-old children being poor or being in the lower half of their class was .08 and .30, respectively.

Thus, as compared to American families that had none of the above three "maternal" risk factors, the existence of which placed new American families in 1990 at a decided disadvantage. Complicating this situation is the fact that these factors do not exist with equal probability across American racial/ethnic groups. Approximately one third (33%) of the new European American families in 1990 had one or more of these three risk factors present, whereas 78% of the new African American families and nearly as many (69%) of the new Latino families had one or more of these factors present (Center for the Study of Social Policy, 1993).

DISPROPORTIONATE REPRESENTATION IN DIVERSE FAMILIES

This overrepresentation of African American and Latino families in this risk category is all the more pronounced given the relatively small proportion of such individuals in contemporary America. For instance, it is still the case that European American children under 18 years of age (who are not of Latino background) comprise 69% of all children in the United States. However, Latino children in this age range constitute only 12% of the child population, while African American children in the age range comprise about 15% of the population of America's children (U.S. Department of Commerce, 1993). The levels of representation of these groups in the United States population makes the disproportionate presence of problems associated with poverty all the more striking.

Moore, Morrison, Zaslow, and Glei (1994), in an analysis of data from the National Longitudinal Study of Youth involving an overrepresentation of African American and Latino youth, found that children from families which were on welfare continuously between 1986 and 1991 were more likely to have high levels of behavior problems than was the case for children that were never on welfare and never poor. Moreover, Moore, et al. (1994) found also that children from families that moved off of welfare but did not move out of poverty were also at high risk for behavior problems. In addition, they report that youth from families that were not poor in 1986 but were both poor and on welfare in 1990 had the highest likelihood of behavior problems. Furthermore, poor children are at high risk of dying from violence. Information from the 1993 *Kids Count Data Book* indicates that between 1985 and 1992 the rate of violent deaths to 15- to 19-year-olds increased by 13%; for European-American youth this increased rate was 10%, whereas for African American 15- to 19-year-olds it was 78%.

In turn, if poor children do not die, their life chances often are squandered by school failure, underachievement, and dropout; crime; teenage pregnancy and parenthood; lack of job preparedness; prolonged welfare dependency; and the feelings of despair and hopelessness that pervade the lives of children whose parents have lived in poverty and who see themselves as having little opportunity to do better, that is, to have a life marked by societal respect, achievement, and opportunity (Dryfoos, 1990; Lerner, 1995; Schorr, 1988). To illustrate, as compared to their nonpoor age-mates, poor youth are: 50% more likely to have physical or mental disability; almost twice as likely not to have visited a doctor or dentist in the most recent two years of their lives; 300% more likely to be high school dropouts; and, as noted above, significantly more likely to be victims of violence (Simons et al., 1991). Furthermore, McLoyd and Wilson (1991) and Klerman (1991) find that poor children live at high risk for low self-confidence, conduct problems, depression, peer conflict, and severe health problems.

In short, the societal and cultural conditions that have created and maintained poverty in America, and that have "distributed" it non-randomly among our families, represent a formidable challenge for research—and for interventions that, ideally, should be informed by, if not derived from, research sensitive to the diverse conditions of poverty. Many poor children live in very diverse families or family-

Family Diversity and Family Policy

type settings, for instance, foster care homes, institutions, shelters, other types of placements, or no fixed settings at all and are homeless (Allison, 1993; Huston, 1991). Lack of attention to this contextual variation may lead to an inadequate appreciation of the diverse role of "the family" in poor children's development. In addition, inattention to this contextual variation may also lead to insufficiently differentiated policies and programs pertinent to the family life of poor children.

THE NEED FOR DIVERSITY-SENSITIVE POLICIES PERTINENT TO POVERTY

For example, in the current welfare reform legislation, there is little acknowledgment of the heterogeneity of the welfare population and their diverse needs (this issue is discussed more fully in Chapter 5). There are few provisions for those welfare recipients who are in need of intensive, longer-term assistance in order to move towards becoming self-sufficient. This refusal to recognize the diversity within the poor has resulted in policies that have the potential to increase the adversity for poor children and their families (Morelli & Verhoef, in press; Smith, Fairchild, & Groginsky, 1997).

The need for more diversity-sensitive policies is only underscored when one appreciates the particular risks and resources associated with each minority group. With regard to risks, Native Americans may be used as a case-in-point.

Native Americans, a group which includes American Indians, the Alaskan natives, and the Native Hawaiians, are one of the most overlooked minority populations in the United States. The groups that comprise Native Americans are an indigenous population to the United States. Although these groups are now increasing in numbers, they remain a relatively invisible yet important minority group which is at great risk and in need of more constructive and "tailored" approaches to public policy that are designed to fit their specific individual, social, and cultural characteristics. Among the key risks confronting these groups are:

- Approximately 20% of American Indian births are to women less than age 20, with 0.4% less than 15 years of age; in comparison, 11.0% European American births are to women less than age 20, with 0.2% less than 15 years of age (Indian Health Services, 1995);
- The three leading causes of death among Indians between infancy and age 14 years include accidents, at twice the rate for European Americans of the same age, and congenital anomalies and homicides, at nearly three times the rate for European Americans age (Indian Health Services, 1995);
- The three leading causes of death among Indian youth 15 to 24 years of age are accidents, at over twice the rate for European Americans; suicide, at 2.5 times the rate for European Americans; and homicide, at almost twice the rate for European Americans (Indian Health Services, 1995)
- 50% of Native Hawaiian mothers are under the age of 18 (Office of Hawaiian Affairs, 1994);

- 18% of the Native Hawaiian population have an annual income under $15,000 (Office of Hawaiian Affairs, 1994);
- Native Hawaiians are in the largest ethnic group with families below the poverty level, the largest ethnic group with families on public assistance, and the largest ethnic group with individuals 200% below the poverty level (Office of Hawaiian Affairs, 1994); and
- Native Hawaiian youth have the highest rates of school absenteeism, school drop-outs, and juvenile delinquency in the State of Hawaii (Office of Hawaiian Affairs, 1994).

We may note that poor families rely on relatives and friends to help them provide care for their children more so than is the case among non-poor families (Morelli & Verhoef, in press), a situation that is certainly understandable given the lack of financial resources among the poor to pay for the provision of quality child care. Nevertheless, before policies are designed in light of such differences, it is important to recognize that, within poor families, there are differences in regard to the use made by different ethnic groups of child care provided by friends and relatives. For example, Morelli and Verhoef (in press, p. 9) report that:

> In a study on low income women in California, Mexican-American mothers were reported to ask relatives to care for their infants and toddlers (65%) more often than White (37%) or Chinese-American mothers (43%).

Moreover, while both Chinese American and non-Hispanic White mothers indicated that center care was the ideal form of care for their children, and while African American mothers use center care more frequently than they do family care, Mexican American mothers believed that relative care was best for their children (Morelli & Verhoef, in press).

In short, then, diversity in both risks and resources needs to be considered in the development of policies for our nation's poor families. Not all poor families are the same. Their diversity provides an important source of resiliency again the stressors of poverty.

RESILIENCY AMONG POOR AND MINORITY FAMILIES AND YOUTH

Of course, just as the absence of risk factors does not promise good parenting or freedom from problems of child development, the relatively high presence of such factors among African American and Latino families does not assure that there will be an occurrence of family instability or poor child outcomes. As Werner and Smith (1982, 1992) and more recently Allison (1993), McAdoo (1998a), McCubbin, et al. (1998), and Spencer (1990) have noted, there are numerous "success stories" among families labeled as "at risk," and many parents and children do not therefore "succumb" to the vulnerability that these factors may represent.

Indeed, it is important to recognize the resiliency of poor and, perhaps especially, of poor *minority* families and the youth within them (given their overrepresentation in America among the ranks of the poor; Huston, 1991; Lerner, 1995), and to seek to understand the developmental pathways that produce this resiliency—even in the face of the host of pernicious factors associated with poverty and racism (e.g., McAdoo, 1977, 1998a; McCubbin, et al., 1998; McLoyd, 1994; McLoyd & Wilson, 1991). These perspectives are important in order to counteract:

> Time lost to considering minorities as "deviant" from majority-based norms rather than exploring the often creative adaptations to life-course discontinuities required of minority families to survive and thrive amid unacknowledged societal inconsistencies. . . . The adaptive modes used by both minority parents and their children requires insights not available from traditional paradigms. (Spencer, 1990, p. 267)

The pioneering work of McAdoo (e.g., 1977, 1982, 1993, 1998a) exemplifies Spencer's (1990) point. McAdoo (1998a) notes that:

> As we look at the development of African-American families over the past three to four hundred years, we are increasingly faced with growing problems among these families: isolation from the economic mainstream, public schools that are becoming even more unsuccessful, violence that abounds in our communities, and more children being raised in families by women alone. It is very tempting to move into a problem oriented focus when one looks at African-American families, for the problems that we face are life threatening and overwhelming. Yet one must avoid this orientation as much as possible, for it will force us to focus on the disproportionate representation of families who are in trouble. We need to examine families who are resilient and who have overcome many of the hurdles present in their environment. We will otherwise overlook the families who are making it everyday, although under less than ideal conditions. They are rearing their children to be competent adults who do not resort to violence, some of whom are even excelling. (p. 19)

The results of McAdoo's scholarship illustrate her perspective. She finds that satisfying family life exists in minority families having diverse structures (e.g., single- and dual-parent households), and that protective factors such as faith play important supportive roles even in families where there is a great deal of stress (e.g., single-parent, female head-of-household families; McAdoo, 1998a). Indeed, the strengths that McAdoo identifies as prototypic in ethnically diverse families have religious institutions as a key source. Such sources of resiliency constitute what McAdoo (1982, p. 479) has termed "stress absorbing systems in Black families."

McCubbin, et al. (1998) discuss such stress absorbing, resilient systems in minority families in general, especially those confronting life challenges (such as poverty or racism). They note that aspects of culture and ethnicity such as family ethnic identification, family schemas, and the customs and traditions of the family are important shapers of family functioning, especially in the face of adversity. Using a relational perspective that emphasizes the harmony and interdependence of relationships, mind, body, and spirit, McCubbin, et al. (1998) emphasize that such features of culture and ethnicity impact resiliency within the context of the family system. In other words, family resiliency arises within a system that integrates ethnic identity and status, actions that preserve cultural and ethnic traditions, the community context and the social milieu of the family, and reciprocal relationships within the family and between the family and the social support resources available in the community (McCubbin, et al., 1998)

Any feature of this system can promote family resiliency. For instance, in homes where there is an absent father, a strong mother-child relation can protect youth from risks (e.g., of having a peer group engaged in problem behaviors) and, in turn, constitutes a source of resiliency and positive development among minority youth (Mason, Cauce, Gonzales, & Hiraga, 1994). In addition, family social support promotes adjustment in minority youth and, as well, provides resiliency in the face of negative life events (Cauce, Felner, & Primavera, 1982; Cauce, Hannan, & Sargeant, 1992; Spencer, 1983).

Other contextual factors described by McCubbin, et al. (1998) also provide sources of resiliency for minority families and youth. For instance, social support provided within the school setting, for example by teachers, promotes school competence (Cauce, et al., 1992; Felner, Aber, Primavera, & Cauce, 1985), and particular school-based programs, such as school-based health service provision programs (Robinson, Ruch-Ross, Watkins-Ferrell, & Lightfoot, 1993), can constitute protective factors for youth. In turn, the work environment of parents and the social support provided by parents combine to reduce externalizing problems among African American adolescents (Mason, et al., 1994). Similarly, peer emotional support and reciprocal best friend relationships are linked with school and peer competence among young African American adolescents (Cauce, 1986).

In turn, individual-psychological characteristics of minority youth also provide protective factors in their development. For instance, perceived self-competence is a key attribute of positive development among minority youth (Cauce, 1986). Other self variables—such as aspirations and future perceptions and self-concept/identity development processes—are also sources of resiliency among minority youth (e.g., Matute-Bianchi, 1986; Spencer, 1984, 1987).

In essence, then, there is a rich array of individual and contextual protective factors that promote resiliency and successful, healthy development among poor and minority youth and families. The presence and strength of these "adaptive modes" (Spencer, 1990, p. 267) underscore the view of McLoyd (1990, p. 263) that "it is myopic, costly, and perilous to ignore the cultural, ecological, and structural forces that enhance" the development of poor and minority youth and families.

CONCLUSIONS

There is a need to attend empirically to the diverse manifestation of poverty in different racial and ethnic groups, and to the challenges faced and resources and strengths of these different groups. This breadth of information will afford the development of sufficiently differentiated policies and programs pertinent to the families of poor children.

It may be deemed by some as impolite or impolitic to note that a shortcoming of scientific inquiry is a failure to pay sufficient attention to the diversity of America's families or to the diversity of the people comprising these institutions. However, such lack of sensitivity to human individual and contextual diversity cannot continue. The absence of sensitivity to diversity is, clearly, morally repugnant to many people *and*, at least equally important in this context, such lack of sensitivity is simply bad science (Lerner, 1991, 1998b).

A key basis of this assertion lies in the view of the importance of a focus on diversity found within developmental contextual theory—a key conceptual perspective involved in the systemic understanding of human individual and social structure, function, and change (Lerner, 1998b; Sameroff, 1983; Thelen & Smith, 1998; Wapner & Demick, 1998). It is useful to review the key features of developmental contextualism in order to understand the implications of the study of diversity for the conduct of science—and for the derivation of policies and programs from such scholarship.

3 DEVELOPMENTAL CONTEXTUALISM AND THE DEVELOPMENTAL SYSTEMS PERSPECTIVE

Developmental contextualism (Lerner, 1986, 1991, 1995, 1998b) is an instance of a theoretical orientation to human development termed "developmental systems theory" (Ford & Lerner, 1992; Sameroff, 1983; Thelen & Smith, 1998). Developmental contextualism has its roots in the multidisciplinary and multiprofessional field of home economics (Lerner & Miller, 1993; Miller & Lerner, 1994), a field now labeled family and consumer sciences. In addition, developmental systems theory, generally, and developmental contextualism, more specifically, have emerged within the current study of human development as representing important, and arguably key, theoretical orientations within the field because of their "co-evolution" with the life-span view of human development (Baltes, 1987; Baltes, Lindenberger, & Staudinger, 1998), the life-course study of human development (Elder, 1974, 1980, 1998), and the ecological view of human development (Bronfenbrenner, 1979; Bronfenbrenner & Crouter, 1983; Bronfenbrenner & Morris, 1998).

The life-span developmental perspective extends the study of development across the course of life by conceptualizing the basic process of development as *relational* in character, that is, as involving associations between the developing individual and his or her complex and changing social and physical context, or ecology. The broadest level of this ecology is history. As explained above with regard to family diversity and family policy, embedding change within a historical context provides a temporal perspective to the study of a phenomenon. Linking the changes that characterize lifespan individual development with an ecology that includes temporality focuses scholarship on the degree of *plasticity* (of the potential for systematic change; Lerner, 1984) that may exist across life. In addition, there is a concern with the characteristics of the person and his or her context that may foster continuity or discontinuity in development.

The life course and the human ecological views of human development also take a view of developmental processes as relational in character. The life course perspective significantly extends the analysis of the developmental process beyond the individual by considering the contributions that institutional structure, function, and change make to the person-context relation and, as well, to the experience of both individuals and groups of individuals (cohorts) developing within specific historical periods. For example, people who were children during the economically difficult period of the Great Depression developed differently across their lives than did people who experienced their childhood years in more economically favorable historical periods (Elder, 1974).

In turn, the human ecological perspective provides understanding of the levels, networks, or social systems or subsystems within which person-context relations occur. This perspective provides developmentalists with an understanding of the dynamics of person-context relations occurring within a specific setting (e.g., the home) within which a person develops (a microsystem); the interconnected set of specific systems (e.g., the home, the classroom, the neighborhood) within which the person develops (the mesosystem); the settings (the exosystem) in which the person does not interact (e.g., the workplace of a young child's parent) but wherein developments occur (e.g., the experience of job-related stress) that influence behavior in the micro- or meso-system; and the broad social institutional context (the macrosystem) that, by virtue of its cultural and public policy components, textures social commerce and influences all other systems embedded within it.

For instance, public policies pertinent to the eligibility of adults to receive public assistance for their children (e.g., Aid for Dependent Children), and cultural attitudes about people who receive such welfare support, may result in specific communities placing time limits on an adult's eligibility for welfare and requiring that the person enter either job training or educational programs. The challenges and stressors that a person has in such a program may influence the emotional character of interactions with his/her child, and the child may carry the "residue" of his/her interaction in the home with the parent into the child's interactions with peers in the classroom.

This example of the applicability of the human ecology perspective can be extended by reference to the life-course viewpoint. Here we might consider the effects on cohorts of poor children growing up in a context where major changes in their family life occur as a consequence of a historically significant change in public policy regarding welfare. In turn, the life-span perspective would extend this example still further by asking questions about whether and how the course of personal development was altered as a consequence of the specific changes that occurred in individual-context relations as a consequence the historically non-normative change in public policy.

Clearly, then, there are important interconnections between the life-span, life-course, and the human ecology perspectives. All viewpoints focus on the linkages that exist between changes within a person over the course of his or her life and the changing structure and function of his or her family, peer group, school, workplace, and community setting, which in turn are embedded within policy, cultural, and historical contexts. All viewpoints are concerned with the way in which the pattern or system of these relations shape human development over the course of life. Simply, all perspectives are concerned with the developmental system and, specifically, with development-in-relation-to-context. By providing a theoretical frame for these viewpoints, developmental contextualism offers a means to integrate and further understanding of the dynamic (that is, bidirectional or reciprocal) relations between people and the settings within which they live their lives. It is useful, then, to summarize some of the key components of the developmental contextual perspective.

FEATURES OF DEVELOPMENTAL CONTEXTUALISM

Developmental contextualism takes an integrative approach to the multiple levels of organization presumed to comprise the nature of human life; that is, *"fused"* (Tobach & Greenberg, 1984) *and changing relations* among biological, psychological, and social contextual levels comprise the process of developmental change. Rather than approaching variables from these levels of analysis in either a reductionistic or in a parallel-processing way, the developmental contextual view rests on the idea that variables from these levels of analysis are dynamically interactive—they are reciprocally influential over the course of human ontogeny.

Within developmental contextualism, levels are conceived of as integrative organizations. That is:

> the concept of integrative levels recognizes as equally essential for the purpose of scientific analysis both the isolation of parts of a whole and their integration into the structure of the whole. It neither reduces phenomena of a higher level to those of a lower one, as in mechanism, or describes the higher level in vague nonmaterial terms which are but substitutes for understanding, as in vitalism. Unlike other "holistic" theories, it never leaves the firm ground of material reality. . . . The concept points to the need to study the organizational interrelationships of parts and whole. (Novikoff, 1945, p. 209)

Moreover, Tobach and Greenberg (1984, p. 2) have stressed that:

> the interdependence among levels is of great significance. The dialectic nature of the relationship among levels is one in which lower levels are subsumed in higher levels so that any particular level is an integration of proceeding levels. . . . In the process of integration, or fusion, *new* levels with their own characteristics result.

If the course of human development is the product of the processes involved in the "fusions" (or "dynamic interactions"; Lerner, 1978, 1979, 1984) among integrative levels, then the processes of development are more plastic than often previously believed (cf. Brim & Kagan, 1980). Within this perspective, the context for development is not seen merely as a simple stimulus environment, but rather as an "ecological environment . . . conceived topologically as a nested arrangement of concentric structures, each contained within the next" (Bronfenbrenner, 1979, p. 22) and including variables from biological, psychological, physical and sociocultural levels, all changing interdependently across history (Riegel, 1975, 1976a, 1976b).

The central idea in developmental contextualism is that changing, reciprocal relations (or dynamic interactions) between individuals and the multiple contexts within which they live comprise the essential process of human development (Lerner, 1986; Lerner & Kauffman, 1985). Accordingly, from a developmental contextual perspective, human behavior—including interactions involving the family and other social institutions—is both biological and social (Featherman & Lerner, 1985; Tobach & Schneirla, 1968). In fact, no form of life as we know it comes into existence independent of other life. No animal lives in total isolation from others of its species across its entire life span (Tobach, 1981; Tobach & Schneirla, 1968). Biological survival requires meeting the demands of the environment or, as we note later, attaining a goodness of fit (Chess & Thomas, 1984; Lerner & Lerner, 1983, 1989; Thomas & Chess, 1977) with the context. Because this environment is populated by other members of one's species, adjustment to (or fit with) these other organisms is a requirement of survival (Tobach & Schneirla, 1968).

Human evolution has promoted this link between biological and social functioning (Featherman & Lerner, 1985; Gould, 1977). Early humans were relatively defenseless, having neither sharp teeth nor claws. Coupled with the dangers of living in the open African savannah, where much of early human evolution occurred, group living was essential for survival (Masters, 1978; Washburn, 1961). Therefore, human beings were more likely to survive if they acted in concert with the group than if they acted in isolation. Human characteristics that support social relations (e.g., attachment, empathy) may have helped human survival over the course of its evolution (Hoffman, 1978; Hogan, Johnson, & Emler, 1978; Sahlins, 1976). Thus, for several reasons, humans at all portions of their life spans may be seen as embedded in a social context with which they have important relationships.

It is important to indicate that we may speak of dynamic interactions between individuals and their contexts that pertain to either *social* or *physical* (for instance, biological or physiological) relations. For example, a parent may "demand" attention from a child who does not show it, "lighting" the parent's "short fuse" of tolerance. He or she then scolds the child, who cries, creating remorse in the parent and eliciting soothing behaviors from him or her. The child is calmed, snuggles up to the parent, and now both parties in the relationship show positive emotions and are happy (see Tubman & Lerner, 1994, for data pertinent to such parent-child relationships).

In turn, dynamic interactions involve not only the exchange of "external" social behaviors but also biological or physiological processes. For example, parental religious practices, rearing practices, or financial status may influence the child's diet and nutritional status, health, and medical care. In turn, the contraction of an infectious disease by either parent or child can lead to the other member of the relationship contracting the disease. Moreover, the health and physical status of the child influences the parent's own feelings of well-being, and his or her hopes and aspirations regarding the child (Finkelstein, 1993).

Family Diversity and Family Policy 29

Thus, the child's physiological status and development are not disconnected from his or her behavioral and social context (in this example, parental) functioning, and development (e.g., see Finkelstein, 1993; Ford & Lerner, 1992; Howard, 1978). The inner and outer worlds of the child are fused and dynamically interactive. In addition, of course, the same may be said of the parent and, in fact, of the parent-child relationship. Each of these foci—child, parent, or relationship—is part of a larger, enmeshed *system* of fused relations among the multiple levels which compose the ecology of human life (Bronfenbrenner, 1979).

For instance, both a parent and child are embedded in a broader social network, and each person has reciprocal reactions with this network. This set of relations occurs because both the child and the parent are much more than just people playing only one role in life. As already emphasized, the child may also be a sibling, peer, and student; the parent may also be a spouse, worker, and adult child. All of these networks of relations are embedded within a particular community, society, and culture. And, finally, all of these relations are continually changing across time and history. Simply, for all portions of the system of person-context, or biology-environment, relations envisioned in developmental contextualism, change across time is an integral, indeed inescapable, feature of human life. The developmental contextual view of human development is illustrated in Figure 3.1.

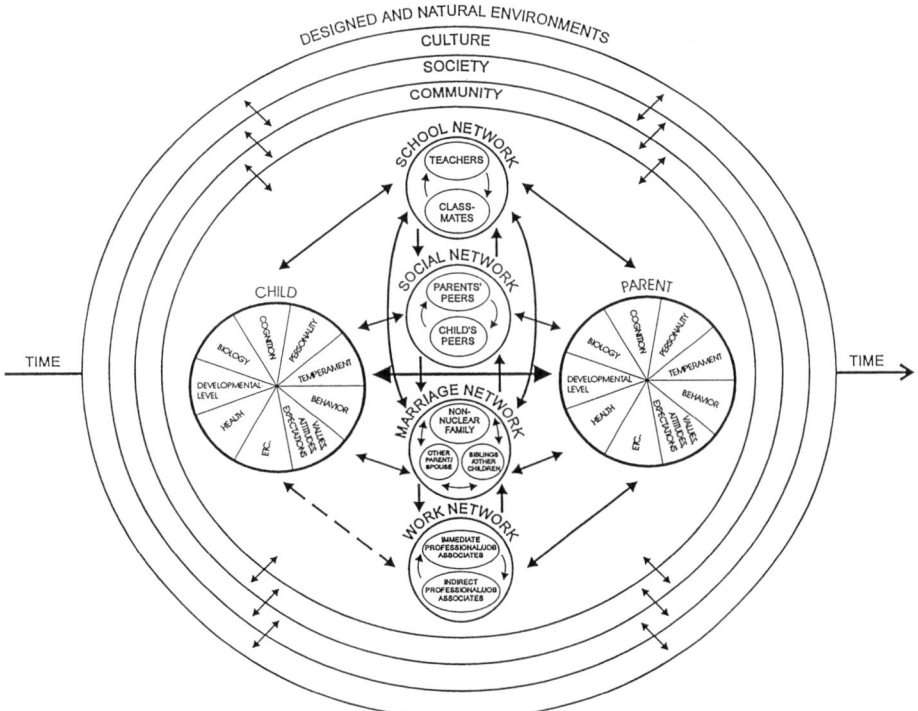

Figure 3.1 *The developmental contextual view of human development*

Within and among each of the networks which is depicted in the figure one may conceive of bidirectional relationships existing among the people populating the network. A child effect may function, in a sense, like a small pebble thrown into a quiet lake. It can prompt a large ripple. In turn, of course, the reverse of this possibility can occur. Events in settings lying far beyond the child-parent relationship can influence it. For instance, the resources in a community for child daycare during the parent's working hours, the laws (e.g., regarding tax exemptions), and the cultural values regarding families who place their infants in daycare, all exert an impact on the quality of the parent-child relationship.

The child-parent relationship, and the social networks in which it is located, are embedded in still larger community, societal, cultural, and historical levels of organization. Time—history—cuts through all the levels of the system. Thus, as with the people populating these social systems, change is always occurring. Diversity within time is created as change across time (across history) introduces variation into all the levels of organization involved in the human development system.

In other words, people develop, the family changes from one having infants and young children, to one having teenagers, to an "empty nest" when the children have left the home of their parents to live elsewhere and very likely to start their own families. Similarly, communities, societies, and cultures change, too (Elder, 1974; Elder, Modell, & Parke, 1993; Garbarino, 1992; Hernandez, 1993). In addition, each of these multiple "levels" is embedded in the natural and human-designed physical ecology, a physical world that of course changes also. Changes at one or more of these levels produce changes in the other levels as well, given their bidirectional connections.

Finally, as we have noted, all changes are embedded in history (Baltes, 1987; Elder, 1974; Elder, et al., 1993), that is, time "cuts through" all levels of organization. As such, the nature of parent-child relations, family life and development, and societal and cultural influences on the child-parent-family system are influenced by both "normative" and "non-normative" historical changes (Baltes, 1987) or, in other words, by "evolutionary" (i.e., gradual) and "revolutionary" (i.e., abrupt; Werner, 1957), historical changes. This system of multiple, interconnected, or "fused" (Tobach & Greenberg, 1984) levels comprises a complete depiction of the integrated organization involved in the developmental contextual view of human development (Lerner, 1986, 1991).

In essence, individuality (diversity), change involving both the individual and the context, and, as a consequence, further individuality, are the essences of human development—of family structure and function—within developmental contextualism. Given that the multiple levels of change involved in person-context relations may involve individuals at any point in their lives, whether they are infants, young children, or adults (and acting in roles such as parents, spouses, or teachers), it is possible to see why a developmental contextual perspective provides a useful frame for studying the diversity of development across the life span.

Indeed, other scholars interested in understanding the development of diverse children, youth, and families have developed models consonant with developmental systems theory. For instance, García Coll, et al. (1996) have formulated an integrative model for studying developmental competencies in minority children. Although they focus on African American and mainland Puerto Rican youth to exemplify the use of the model, García Coll, et al. emphasize that the model is generalizable to other ethnic and minority groups. The conception forwarded by García Coll, et al. builds on McAdoo's (1992) idea that ecological-developmental models may be useful in describing the contexts of diverse youth and families when they are extended to include societal racism, classism, and sexism.

Accordingly, the model developed by García Coll, et al. (1996) includes:

- Social position variables, such as race, social class, ethnicity, and gender;
- Problematic social and cultural phenomena, such as racism, prejudice, discrimination, and oppression;
- Segregation, in residential, economic, social, and psychological domains;
- Promoting/inhibiting environments, involving schools, neighborhoods, and the health care system;
- Adaptive cultural phenomena, such as traditions and cultural legacies, economic and political histories, migration and acculturation, and current contextual demands;
- Child characteristics, such as age, temperament, health status, biological factors, and physical characteristics;
- Family variables, such as structure and roles, family values, beliefs, and goals, racial socialization, and socioeconomic status; and
- Developmental competencies, with regard to cognition, social, emotional, and linguistic functioning, biculturalism, and coping with racism.

Taylor Gibbs and Huang (1998) present a model for psychological interventions with culturally diverse youth that also is consistent with developmental systems theory. They approach intervention with diverse youth within the context of an integrative and interactive developmental-ecological framework that focuses explicitly on culture. The model specifies the role of ethnic variation and context in the design of effective programs for youth. Thus, Taylor Gibbs and Huang stress the significance of the family, peer group, school, and community in the design of treatments for children and adolescents. The importance of this multilevel, integrative approach to intervention is illustrated in regard to children and adolescents from Chinese American, Japanese American, Native American, African American, Mexican American, Puerto Rican, and Southeast Asian backgrounds. In addition, the use of the model for interventions for biracial adolescents is illustrated.

As noted at the beginning of this chapter, development contextualism is an instance of a more general theoretical view of human development—developmental systems—that provides understanding not only of individual diversity but, as well, of family diversity. The features of developmental systems theory are useful also to understand.

THE IMPORTANCE OF DEVELOPMENTAL SYSTEMS THEORY FOR RESEARCH AND APPLICATION PERTINENT TO FAMILY DIVERSITY AND FAMILY POLICY

One reason that the families and children of America face the singular set of risks confronting them is that for too long scholars followed a model that treated the problems of youth development as issues of "only" applied concern—and thus of secondary scientific interest. Not only did this model separate basic science from application but, as well, it disembedded the developing person from his or her context and treated the variables that were presumed to influence behavior and development as if they could be studied and understood in a decontextualized, reductionistic manner.

Thus, the conception of developmental process in this model often involved causal splits between individual and context, between organism and environment, or—most generally—between nature and nurture (Gottlieb, 1997). Theories based on this model emphasized either predetermined organismic bases of development, for instance, as in attachment theory (e.g., Bowlby, 1969); ethological theory (e.g., Lorenz, 1965); behavioral genetics (e.g., Plomin, 1986); psychoanalytic theory (e.g., Freud, 1954), and neo-psychoanalytic theory (e.g., A. Freud, 1969; Erikson, 1968); or environmental, reductionistic, and mechanistic bases of behavior and behavior change (e.g., Bijou & Baer, 1961, 1965; Gerwitz & Stingle, 1968).

Other theories stressed more of an interaction between organismic and environmental sources of development (e.g., Piaget, 1950, 1970). Nevertheless, there remained in the discipline a presupposition that there were two distinct sources of development, that is, that there was a split between organism and environment. As such, it was the role of theory to explain the contributions of these two separate domains of reality to human development (Overton, 1998).

In short, then, scholars studying human development have for too long used a theoretical model of human development that was not able to be deployed usefully in understanding the relational nature of development (Overton, 1998) and of the synthesis between basic and applied concerns legitimated by relational models of development (Lerner, 1995, 1996, 1998b; Lerner, et al., 1994). However, these non-relational "split" theories of human development are, today, no longer the predominant ones in the disciplines involved in the study of adolescence (Cairns, 1998; Dixon & Lerner, 1999; Lerner, 1998a). Today, cutting-edge theoretical and empirical scholarship about human development that uses dynamic systems models to understand and enhance the trajectory of change across the life span (Lerner, 1998a)

CONTEMPORARY DEVELOPMENTAL SYSTEMS MODELS OF HUMAN DEVELOPMENT

The stress in contemporary developmental theories is on a "healing" of the nature-nurture split (Gottlieb, 1997), and on accounting for how the integrated developmental system functions, i.e., for understanding probabilistic epigenesis.

Gottlieb (1997, p. 90) defined this process as being *"characterized by an increase of complexity or organization—that is, the emergence of new structural and functional properties and competencies—at all levels of analysis* (molecular, subcellular, cellular, organismic) *as a consequence of horizontal and vertical coactions among its parts, including organism-environment coactions."*

As such, the forefront of contemporary developmental theory and research is represented by theories of process—of how structures function and how functions are structured over time (Lerner, 1996, 1998b). For example, most contemporary research about human development is associated with theoretical ideas stressing that the dynamics of individual-context relations provide the bases of behavior and developmental change (see, too, Lerner, 1986, 1998a). Indeed, even models that try to separate biological or, more particularly, genetic, influences on an individual's development from contextual ones are at pains to (retro)fit their approach into a more dynamic systems perspective (e.g., as found in Ford & Lerner, 1992; Gottlieb, 1992; Thelen & Smith, 1994; Wapner, 1993).

In emphasizing that systematic and successive change (i.e., development) is associated with alterations in the dynamic relations among structures from multiple levels of organization, the scope of contemporary developmental theory and research is not limited by (or, perhaps better, confounded by an inextricable association with) a unidimensional portrayal of the developing person (e.g., the person seen from the vantage point of only cognitions, or emotions, or stimulus-response connections, or genetic imperatives; for example, see Piaget, 1970; Freud, 1949; Bijou & Baer, 1961; and Rowe, 1994, respectively). Rather, the power of the contemporary stress on processes of dynamic person-context relations is the "design criteria" imposed on research, method, and application pertinent to the study of any content area or dimension of the developing person. This power is constituted by four interrelated, and in fact "fused" (Tobach & Greenberg, 1984), assumptive dimensions of contemporary theories of human development (Lerner, 1998b). Accordingly, it is useful to discuss these dimensions in order to illuminate the key theoretical and methodological (e.g., research design and measurement) issues pertinent to understanding how biological, psychological, and contextual processes combine to promote behavior and development across the life span.

Change and Relative Plasticity

Contemporary theories stress that the focus of developmental understanding must be on systematic *change* (Ford & Lerner, 1992). This focus is required because of the belief that the potential for change exists across the life span (e.g., Baltes, 1987). Although it is also assumed that systemic change is not limitless (e.g., it is constrained by both past developments and by contemporary contextual conditions), contemporary theories stress that *relative plasticity* exists across life—although the magnitude of this plasticity may vary across ontogeny (Lerner, 1984).

There are important implications of relative plasticity for the application of developmental science. For instance, the presence of relative plasticity legitimates a proactive search across the life span for characteristics of people and their contexts that, together, can influence the design of policies and programs promoting positive development (Birkel, Lerner, and Smyer, 1989; Fisher & Lerner, 1994; Lerner & Hood, 1986).

Relationism and the Integration of Levels of Organization

Contemporary theories stress that the bases for change—and for both plasticity and constraints in development—lie in the relations that exist among the multiple levels of organization that comprise the substance of human life (Ford & Lerner, 1992; Schneirla, 1957; Tobach, 1981). These levels range from the inner biological level, through the individual/psychological level and the proximal social relational level (e.g., involving dyads, peer groups, and nuclear families), to the sociocultural level (including key macro-institutions such as educational, public policy, governmental, and economic systems), and the natural and designed physical ecologies of human development (Bronfenbrenner, 1979; Riegel, 1975). These levels are structurally and functionally integrated, thus requiring a systems view of the levels involved in human development (Ford & Lerner, 1992; Sameroff, 1983; Thelen & Smith, 1994).

As we have noted above, developmental contextualism (Lerner, 1986, 1991, 1995) is one instance of such a developmental systems perspective, and promotes a *relational* unit of analysis as a requisite for developmental analysis (Lerner, 1991). Variables associated with any level of organization exist (are structured) in relation to variables from other levels. The qualitative and quantitative dimensions of the function of any variable are shaped as well by the relations that variable has with ones from other levels. Unilevel units of analysis (or the components of, or elements in, a relation) are not an adequate target of developmental analysis; rather, the relation itself—the interlevel linkage—should be the focus of such analysis (Lerner, 1991; Riegel, 1975).

Relationism and integration have a clear implication for unilevel theories of development. At best, such theories are severely limited and inevitably provide a non-veridical depiction of development, due to their focus on what are essentially main effects embedded in higher-order interactions (e.g., see Walsten, 1990). At worst, such theories are neither valid nor useful. Accordingly neither biogenic theories (e.g., genetic reductionistic conceptions such as behavioral genetics or sociobiology; Freedman, 1979; Rowe, 1994), psychogenic theories (e.g., behavioristic or functional analysis models; Bijou, 1976; Bijou & Baer, 1961), nor sociogenic theories (e.g., "social mold" conceptions of socialization; for example, Homans, 1961; and see Hartup, 1978, for a review) provide adequate theoretical frames for understanding human development). Simply, neither nature nor nurture theories provide adequate conceptualizations of human development (cf. Hirsch, 1970). For instance, theories that stress critical periods of development (e.g., Bowlby, 1969; Erikson, 1959; Lorenz, 1965), that is, periods of ontogeny constrained by biology (e.g., by genetics or maturation), are seen from the perspective of theories that stress relationism and integration as conceptually flawed (and empirically counterfactual).

Moreover, many nature-nurture interaction theories also fall short in this regard, treating nature- and nurture-variables as separable entities, and viewing their connection in manners analogous to the interaction term in an analysis of variance (e.g., Bijou, 1976; Erikson, 1959; Rowe, 1994; cf. Gollin, 1981; Hebb, 1970; Walsten, 1990). The cutting-edge of contemporary theory moves beyond the simplistic division of sources of development into nature-related and nurture-related variables or processes, instead the multiple levels of organization within the ecology of human development are seen as part of an inextricably fused developmental system.

Historical Embeddedness and Temporality

The relational units of analysis of concern in contemporary theories are understood as change units (Lerner, 1991). The change component of these units derives from the ideas that all of the above-noted levels of organization involved in human development are embedded in history, integrated with historical change (Elder, 1980; Elder, et al., 1993). Relationism and integration mean that no level of organization functions as a consequence of its own isolated activity (Tobach, 1981). Each level functions as a consequence of its fusion (structural integration) with other levels (Tobach & Greenberg, 1984). History—change over time—is incessant and continuous, and it is a level of organization that is fused with all other levels. This linkage means that change is a necessary, inevitable feature of variables from all levels of organization (Baltes, 1987; Lerner, 1984). It also means that the structure, as well as the function, of variables changes over time.

Indeed, at the biological level of organization one prime set of structural changes across history is subsumed under the concept of evolution (Gould, 1977; Lewontin, 1981; Lewontin, Rose, & Kamin, 1984). Of course, the concept of evolution can be applied also to functional changes (Darwin, 1872; Gottlieb, 1992). In turn, at more macro levels of organization many of the historically-linked changes in social and cultural institutions or products are evaluated in the context of discussions of the concept of progress (Nisbet, 1980). The continuity of change that constitutes history can lead to both intraindividual (or, more generally, intralevel) continuity or discontinuity in development, depending on the rate, scope, and particular substantive component of the developmental system at which change is measured (Brim & Kagan, 1980; Lerner, 1986, 1988; Lerner & Tubman, 1989). Thus, continuity at one level of analysis may be coupled with discontinuity at another level; quantitative continuity or discontinuity may be coupled with qualitative continuity or discontinuity within and across levels; and continuity or discontinuity can exist in both the processes involved in (or the "explanations" of) developmental change and the features, depictions, or outcomes (i.e., the "descriptions") of these processes (Cairns & Hood, 1983; Lerner, 1986).

These patterns of within-person change pertinent to continuity and discontinuity can result in either constancy or variation in the rates at which different individuals develop with regard to a particular substantive domain of development. Thus, any pattern of intraindividual change can be combined with any instance of interindividual differences in within-person change (i.e., with any pattern of stability or instability; Lerner, 1986; Lerner & Tubman, 1989). In other words, continuity-discontinuity is a dimension of intraindividual change and is distinct from, and independent of, stability-instability—which involves between-person change, and is, therefore, a group, and not an individual, concept (Baltes & Nesselroade, 1973; Lerner, 1986).

In sum, since historical change is continuous, temporality is infused in all levels of organization. This infusion may be associated with different patterns of continuity and discontinuity across people. The potential array of such patterns has implications for understanding the importance of human diversity.

The Limits of Generalizability, Diversity, and Individual Differences

The temporality of the changing relations among levels of organization means that changes that are seen within one historical period (or time of measurement), and/or with one set of instances of variables from the multiple levels of the ecology of human development, may not be seen at other points in time (Baltes, Reese, & Nesselroade, 1977; Bronfenbrenner, 1979). What is seen in one data set is only an instance of what does or could exist. Accordingly, contemporary theories focus on diversity—of people, relations, settings, and times of measurement (Lerner, 1991, 1995).

Individual differences within and across all levels of organization are seen as having core substantive significance in the understanding of human development (Baltes, 1987; Lerner, 1991, 1995). Diversity is the exemplary illustration of the presence of relative plasticity in human development (Lerner, 1984). Diversity is also the best evidence that exists of the potential for change in the states and conditions of human life (Brim & Kagan, 1980).

Moreover, the individual structural and functional characteristics of a person constitute an important source of his or her development (Lerner, 1982; Lerner & Busch-Rossnagel, 1981). The individuality of each person promotes variation in the fusions he or she has with the levels of organization within which the person is embedded. For instance, the distinct actions or physical features of a person promote differential actions (or reactions) in others toward him or her (Lerner, 1987). These differential actions, which constitute feedback to the person, shape at least in part further change in the person's characteristics of individuality (Schneirla, 1957; Lerner & Lerner, 1989). For example, the changing match, congruence, or goodness-of-fit between the developmental characteristics of the person and his or her context provide a basis for consonance or dissonance in the ecological milieu of the person. The dynamic nature of this interaction constitutes a source of variation in positive and negative outcomes of developmental change (Lerner & Lerner, 1983; Thomas & Chess, 1977).

The major assumptive dimensions of contemporary theories of human development—systematic change and relative plasticity; relationism and integration; embeddedness and temporality; generalizability limits and diversity—are very much intertwined facets of a common paradigmatic core. And, as is also the case with the levels of organization that are integrated to form the substance of developmental change, the assumptive dimensions form the corpus of superordinate developmental systems views of human development (Ford & Lerner, 1992), e.g., developmental contextualism. As is the case with the several defining features of the life-span developmental perspective, which—according to Baltes (1987)—need to be considered as an integrated whole, the assumptive dimensions of contemporary developmental theories need to be appreciated simultaneously. Such appreciation is required to understand the breadth, scope, and implications for research and application of this "family" of conceptual frameworks—to development across the life span and, of particular relevance here, to research and application pertinent to individual and family development.

APPLYING DEVELOPMENTAL SYSTEMS: PERSPECTIVES ABOUT RESEARCH AND APPLICATION

Developmental systems models stress that reciprocal changes among levels of organization are both products and producers of the reciprocal changes within levels. For example, over time, parents' "styles" of behavior and rearing influence children's personality and cognitive functioning and development. In turn, the interactions between personality and cognition constitute an emergent "characteristic" of human individuality that affects parental behaviors and styles and the quality of family life (e.g., Lerner, 1982; Lerner & Busch-Rossnagel, 1981; Lerner, Castellino, et al., 1995; Lewis, 1997).

Not only do we believe that a focus on process and, particularly, on the process involved in the changing relations between individuals and their contexts, is at the cutting-edge of contemporary developmental theory and, as such, is the predominant conceptual frame for research in the study of human development (Lerner, 1998a), but we believe as well that these theoretical and empirical orientations represent the key frame for much of the research in the study of family and individual diversity. For example, most contemporary research about human development is associated with theoretical ideas stressing that the dynamics of individual-context relations provide the bases of behavior and developmental change (see, too, Lerner, 1986, 1995, 1996, 1998b; Lerner, Petersen, & Brooks-Gunn, 1991). Thus, in emphasizing that systematic and successive change (i.e., development) is associated with alterations in the dynamic relations among structures from multiple levels of organization, the scope of contemporary developmental theory and research is not limited by (or, perhaps better, confounded by an inextricable association with) a unidimensional portrayal of the developing person (e.g., the person seen from the vantage point of only cognitions, or emotions, or stimulus-response connections, or genetic imperatives; for example, see Piaget, 1970; Freud, 1949; Bijou & Baer, 1961; and Rowe, 1994, respectively). Rather, the power of the contemporary stress on processes of dynamic person-context relations is the focus on process imposed on research, about any content area or dimension of the developing adolescent and on applications to policies and programs (e.g., Bronfenbrenner, McClelland,

Wethington, Moen, & Ceci, 1996; Bronfenbrenner & Morris, 1998; Fisher & Lerner, 1994; Kendall, Chansky, & Kortlander, 1994; McAdoo, 1998a, 1998b, 1999). Emphases in such applications are based on determining the relations between individuals and their settings, rather than on changing either youth or context per se.

These conceptual and empirical orientations represent the essential approaches within the preponderant majority of theoretically derived scholarship in the contemporary study of human development. For instance, to gain understanding of how variations in adolescent-context relations may influence actual or to-be-actualized developmental trajectories, researchers may act to change either the proximal and/or distal natural ecology (e.g., Bronfenbrenner, et al., 1996). Evaluation of the outcomes of such contextual changes—which, in effect, constitute interventions into the course of human development is a means to bring data to bear on theoretical issues pertinent to changing person-context relations and, more specifically, on the plasticity in human development that may exist, or that may be capitalized on through interventions, to enhance human life (Lerner, 1995).

A developmental systems perspective involves the study of active people providing a source, across the life span, of their individual developmental trajectories. This development occurs through the dynamic interactions people experience with the specific characteristics of the changing contexts within which they are embedded (Brandtstädter, 1998). This stress on the dynamic relation between the individual and his or her context results in the recognition that a synthesis of perspectives from multiple disciplines is needed to understand the multilevel (e.g., person, family, and community) integrations involved in human development. In addition, to understand the basic process of human development—the process of change involved in the relations between individuals and contexts—both descriptive and explanatory research must be conducted within the actual ecology of people's lives.

In the case of explanatory studies, such investigations, by their very nature, constitute intervention research. The role of the developmental researcher conducting explanatory research is to understand the ways in which variations in person-context relations account for the character of human developmental trajectories, life paths that are enacted in the "natural laboratory" of the "real world." Therefore, to gain understanding of how theoretically relevant variations in person-context relations may influence developmental trajectories, the researcher may introduce policies and/or programs as "experimental manipulations" of the proximal and/or distal natural ecology. Evaluations of the outcomes of such interventions then become a means to bring data to bear on theoretical issues pertinent to person-context relations and, more specifically, on the plasticity in human development that may exist, or that may be capitalized on, to enhance human life (Csikszentmihalyi & Rathunde, 1998; Lerner, 1984). In other words, a key theoretical issue for explanatory research in human development is the extent to which changes—in the multiple, fused levels of organization comprising human life—can alter the structure and/or function of behavior and development.

Life itself is, of course, an intervention. The accumulation of the specific roles and events a person experiences across the life span—involving normative age-graded events, normative history-graded events, and nonnormative events (Baltes, Reese, & Lipsitt, 1980; Baltes et al., 1998)—alters each person's developmental trajectory in a manner that would not have occurred had another set of roles and events been experienced. The interindividual differences in intraindividual change that exist as a consequence of these naturally occurring interventions attest to the magnitude of the systematic changes in structure and function—the plasticity—that characterize human life.

Explanatory research is necessary, however, to understand what variables, from what levels of organization, are involved in particular instances of plasticity that have been seen to exist. In addition, such research is necessary to determine what instances of plasticity may be created by science or society. In other words, explanatory research is needed to ascertain the extent or limits of human plasticity (Baltes, 1987; Baltes et al., 1998; Lerner, 1984). From a developmental systems perspective, the conduct of such research may lead the scientist to alter the natural ecology of the person or group he or she is studying. Such research may involve proximal and/or distal variations in the context of human development (Lerner & Ryff, 1978); in either case, these manipulations constitute theoretically guided alterations of the roles and events a person or group experiences at, or over, a portion of the life span.

These alterations are, then, interventions—planned attempts to alter the system of person-context relations that constitute the basic process of change. They are conducted in order to ascertain the specific bases, or to test the limits, of particular instances of human plasticity (Baltes, 1987; Baltes & Baltes, 1980; Baltes et al., 1998). These interventions are a researcher's attempt to substitute designed person-context relations for naturally occurring ones in an effort to understand the process of changing person-context relations that provides the basis of human development. In short, basic research in human development is intervention research (Lerner et al., 1994).

Accordingly, the cutting edge of theory and research in human development lies in the application of the conceptual and methodological expertise of human development scientists to the natural ontogenetic laboratory of the real world. Multilevel—and hence, multivariate—and longitudinal research methods must be used by scholars from multiple disciplines to derive, from theoretical models of person-context relations, programs of "applied research." These endeavors must involve the design, delivery, and evaluation of interventions aimed at enhancing—through scientist-introduced variation—the course of human development (Birkel, Lerner, & Smyer, 1989).

Relationism and contextualization have brought to the fore of scientific, intervention, and policy concerns some issues that are pertinent to the functional import of diverse instances of person-context interactions. Examples are studies of the effects of maternal employment, marital disruption, or single-parent families, on infant, child, and young adolescent development; the importance of quality day care, variation in school structure and function, and neighborhood resources and programs for the immediate and long-term development in children of healthy physical, psychological, and social characteristics; and the effects of peer group norms and behaviors, risk behaviors, and economic resources on the healthy development of children and youth.

As a result of greater study of the actual contexts within which children and parents live, behavioral and social scientists have shown increasing appreciation of the diversity of patterns of individual and family development that exist, and that comprise the range of human structural and functional characteristics. Such diversity—involving racial, ethnic, gender, national, and cultural variation—has, to the detriment of the knowledge base in human development, not been a prime concern of empirical analysis (Fisher, Jackson, & Villarruel, 1998; Hagen, Paul, Gibb, & Wolters, 1990).

Yet, for several reasons, this diversity must become a key focus of concern in the study of human development. Diversity of people and their settings means that one cannot assume that general rules of development either exist for, or apply in the same way to, all children and families (Fisher & Brennan, 1992; Fisher & Tryon, 1990; Lerner, 1988; Lerner & Tubman, 1989). As discussed more fully in Chapter 4, this is not to say that general features of human development do not exist, or that descriptive research documenting such characteristics is not an important component of past, present, and future scholarship. However, the lawful individuality of human behavior and development means that one should not make a priori assumptions that characteristics identified in one group, or even in several groups, exist or function in the same way in another group. Moreover, even when common characteristics are identified in diverse groups, we cannot be certain that the individual or unique attributes of each group—even if they account for only a small proportion of the variance in the respective groups' functioning—are not of prime import for understanding the distinctive nature of the groups' development or for planning key components of policies or programs (i.e., for planning "services") designed for the groups.

As we argue in Chapter 8, a new research agenda that focuses on diversity and context while at the same time attending to commonalties of individual development, family changes, and the mutual influences between the two is necessary. Diversity should be placed at the fore of our research agenda. Then, with a knowledge of individuality, we can determine empirically the parameters of commonality, of interindividual generalizability. We should no longer make a priori assumptions about the existence of generic developmental laws or the primacy of such laws, even if they are found to exist, in providing the key information about the life of a given person or group. Integrated multidisciplinary and developmental research devoted to the study of diversity and context must be moved to the fore of scholarly concern.

In sum, then, the developmental systems perspective that characterizes contemporary developmental theory serves as a frame not only for the advancement of understanding about human development but, as well, for enhancing the development of individuals and families whose quality of life is being challenged by both normative developmental problems and risks associated with the current historical moment (e.g., see Bronfenbrenner et al., 1996). This developmental systems perspective, then, in synthesizing basic and applied scientific activities pertinent to the human life course, constitutes a model through which researchers can pursue the cutting-edge of scholarship in their field and, at the same time, conduct work that serves the interests of those sectors of society concerned primarily with addressing the problems of America's youth through programs and policies (Fisher & Lerner, 1994). If so, then such scholarship may become a means through which academe can contribute effectively to community-based attempts to promote positive youth development (Lerner & Simon, 1998a).

ENHANCING APPLIED DEVELOPMENTAL SCIENCE ACROSS THE LIFE SPAN

The future scholarly and societal significance of the study of individual and family development lies in application of developmental science, that is, in building a scientific enterprise that works to help envision, enact, and sustain effective policies and programs promoting the positive development of people across the life span (Zigler & Finn-Stevenson, 1992). Such a focus of scholarship is, on the one hand, a logical and—if judged by the above noted trends in the theoretical foci of the human development field—inevitable outcome of the growth and progress we have experienced as a scientific community (Cairns, 1998; Zigler & Finn-Stevenson, 1992). On the other hand, the four key sets of conceptual themes involved in contemporary developmental systems theories lead us to embrace a focus on: (a) ecologically embedded research, (b) testing our notions of person-context relational systems, and (c) relative plasticity, in order to appraise whether theoretically predicated changes in the nature and course of the relations children have with the proximal and distal features of their context can alter in salutary ways the trajectories of their development. In other words, the concepts of development embraced in our field lead us to test our theories through intervention/action research. We will return to this point in Chapter 8. Here, it may suffice to indicate that we believe that within the field of scholarship about human development, basic research and applied research are synthetic, indivisible endeavors.

Developmental systems perspective leads us to recognize that if we are to have an adequate and sufficient science of child development, we must integratively study individual and contextual levels of organization in a relational and temporal manner (Bronfenbrenner, 1974; McAdoo, 1999; Zigler & Finn-Stevenson, 1992). Anything less will not constitute adequate science. And if we are to serve America's children and families through our science, if we are to help develop successful policies and programs through our scholarly efforts, then we must accept nothing less than the integrative temporal and relational model of the child that is embodied in the developmental systems perspective forwarded in contemporary theories of human development.

Through its research, our field has an opportunity to serve both scholarship and the communities, families, and people of our world. By integrating policies and programs sensitive to the diversity of our communities and our people, by combining the assets of our scholarly traditions with the strengths of our people, we can improve on the often-cited idea of Kurt Lewin (1943) that there is nothing as practical as a good theory. We can, through the application of our science to serving our world's diverse citizens, actualize the idea that there is nothing of greater value to society than a science devoted to using its scholarship to improve the life chances of all people.

We believe there is great substantive importance for focusing on the diversity of individuals and families in applied developmental science, perhaps especially when such work is directed to engaging the policy making process. We discuss the bases of our view in Chapter 4.

4 ENGAGING PUBLIC POLICY: THE SUBSTANTIVE IMPORTANCE OF DIVERSITY

There are several reasons why diversity should become a key focus of concern in the study of human development (Lerner, 1991, 1992, 1998) and in the applications of such scholarship to the policy making process. As noted by McLoyd (1994), by 1990 about 25% of all Americans had African, Asian, Latino, or Native American ancestry. Moreover, the proportion of Americans from other than European backgrounds will continue to grow; for example, more than 80% of legal immigrants to America continue to be from non-European backgrounds (Barringer, 1991; McAdoo, 1998a, 1998b, 1999).

Furthermore, McLoyd (1994) notes that higher fertility rates among minority groups continue to contribute to the increasing proportion of the American population that is comprised by groups that are now considered minorities. However, by the end of this century the Latino population in America will increase by about 21%, the Asian American population by about 22%, and the African American population by about 12%; however, the European American population will grow by only about 2% (Barringer, 1991; McLoyd, 1994; Wetzel, 1987). The American and Alaskan Native population is growing at an estimated rate of more than 2.0% per year, and between 1980 and 1990, the American Indian population grew 54% (Office of Special Education, Department of Education, 1995). Accordingly, by about the year 2000, approximately 33% of all American children and youth will be from "minority" groups and, in some states (e.g., California, Texas, and New Mexico) the majority of youth are already, or by the year 2000 will be, from "minority" groups (Dryfoos, 1990; Henry, 1990; McLoyd, 1994).

Given these demographic trends, it is not appropriate—and, in fact, it might be disastrous for the future health and welfare of America—to ignore in our scientific research or outreach the diversity of America's children. As stressed by McLoyd (1994, pp. 59-60):

> In view of these demographic changes, rendering minority children virtually invisible in the annals of knowledge about the conditions that facilitate and disrupt development is indefensible ethically. That some of the most pressing problems now facing America affect, disproportionately, children and youth from ethnic minority backgrounds makes it all the more so. It is also inimical to the

> long-term self-interests of the nation because minority youth's fraction of the total youth population is increasing precisely at a time when the proportion of youth in the total population is dwindling. . . . Consequently, the proportion of youths in the total population will continue to fall, reaching a low of 13% in 1996, down from 19% in 1980. The implications of this trend are far-reaching. The decline in the number of youth, and ultimately, the number of entrants into the labor force, means that the ratio of workers to retirees will shrink. The economic well-being of the nation will depend even more than at present on its ability to enhance the intellectual and social skills of all its youth, as these will be crucial for maximum productivity in the workplace.

Moreover, evidence for the presence and substantive and societal importance of individual diversity is coupled with similar information relevant to the significance of contextual variation in human development. We have considered the nature of contemporary and historical diversity in the structure and function of the American family. However, examples exist of the significance of contextual variation for human development other than those pertaining specifically to the family. A key instance here, especially insofar as it pertains to building policies and programs that address the problems of youth developing in poor or low-income families and neighborhoods (Lerner, 1995), involves the needs and assets of communities.

DIVERSITY IN THE CHARACTERISTICS OF POOR COMMUNITIES

Given the historical record in child development research of insensitivity to the general environment, or context, within which children develop (Bronfenbrenner, 1977, 1979; Hagen, et al., 1990), it is not surprising that little attention has been paid to the variation that exists *within* any given setting. After all, if the context in general has not been of particular concern to child development researchers, then it is understandable that even less interest has been shown about the potential importance for development of either variation across or variation within contexts (Elder, et al., 1993).

One instance of a lack of attention to important contextual diversity occurs in respect to poor or low income communities (Kretzmann & McKnight, 1993; McKnight & Kretzmann, 1993). Often these neighborhoods are seen to be exclusively characterized by needs and deficits. For instance, McKnight and Kretzmann (1993) note that such settings may be often aptly characterized as being comprised of slum housing, crime gangs, drug abuse, and the other neighborhood needs or deficits depicted in the "map" presented in Figure 4.1.

However, while these needs are in fact often all present in such communities, a sole focus on such problems will result in a significant underestimation of the capacity of the community for marshaling the human, and even fiscal, resources necessary for the design and implementation of programs promoting positive

Family Diversity and Family Policy 45

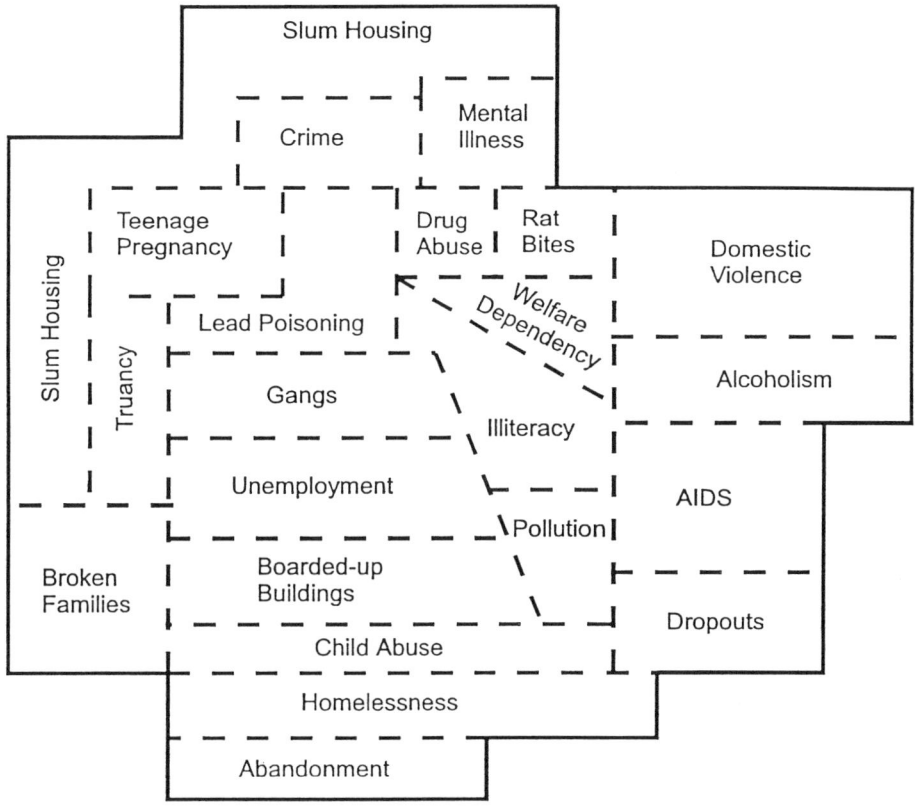

Figure 4.1 *An example of a "neighborhood needs" map (McKnight & Kretzmann, 1993)*

features of human development. McKnight and Kretzmann (1993) note that poor neighborhoods have assets such as cultural and religious organizations, public schools, citizen associations, and the other assets depicted in the "map" presented in Figure 4.2.

For example, looking at pre-existing organizations can be a significant resource for promoting resiliency and protective factors in resource limited poor communities. Cultural organizations can facilitate enculturation, the process by which individuals learn about and identify with their traditional ethnic culture (Zimmerman, Ramirez, Washienko, Walter, & Dyer, 1998). Cultural awareness and understanding is a lifelong developmental process and can increase cultural pride and self-esteem, as well as influence other dimensions of a person's life including spirituality, religion, family, and the community. Phinney and Chavira (1992) and Zimmerman, et al. (1998) find that enculturation and participation in cultural activities can improve psychological well-being and act as protective factors against risky and/or problematic behavior among African American, Latino, Asian American, and Native American youth.

Assets such as cultural organizations that promote ethnic pride within the community and that are under the neighborhood's control need to be recognized by researchers and outreach scholars as resources that can enhance these communities. Unless attention is paid to such strengths, that is, to the fact that there is diversity involving *both* needs and resources, only a deficit model of poor communities will be available to inform ideas for policies and programs pertinent to the people living in such settings. As such, both research and outreach will underestimate the human capital that exists and that may be enhanced in poor and low income communities.

In sum, diversity of people and their settings means that one cannot assume that general rules of development either exist for, or apply in the same way to, all children and families. Moreover, one cannot assume, even if only small portions of the total variance in human behavior and development reflect variance that is unique

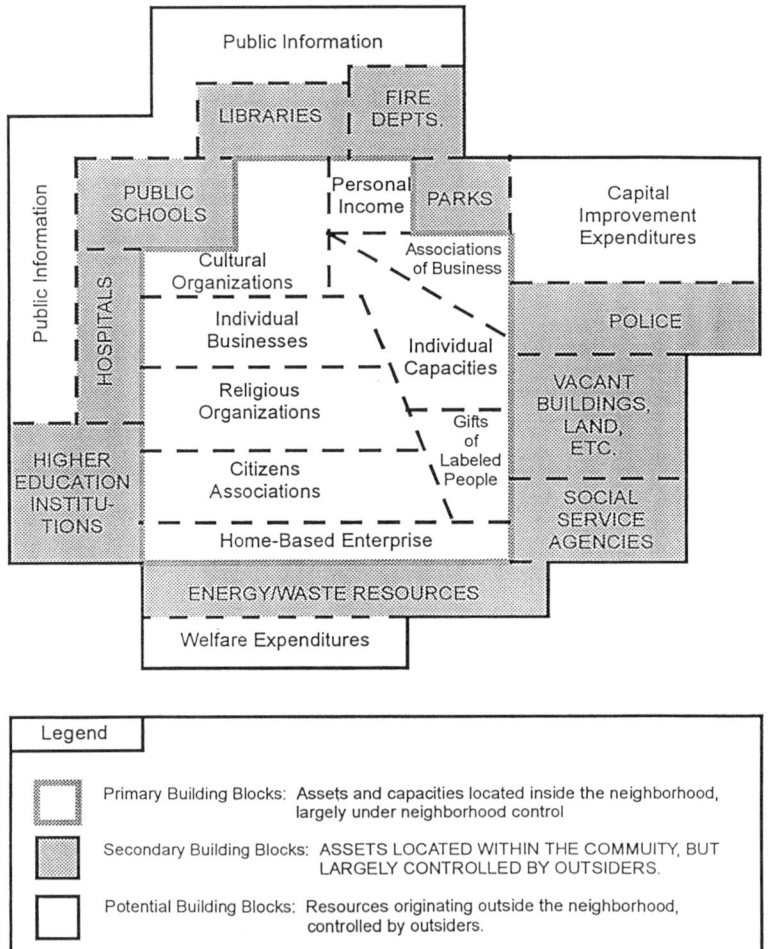

Figure 4.2 *An example of a "neighborhoods assets" map (McKnight & Kretzmann, 1993)*

to an individual or group, that this non-shared variance is not the most salient information we have when attempting to understand or enhance the quality of the lives for the person or group. Accordingly, a new research agenda is promoted. This agenda would focus on diversity and context while at the same time attending to individual development, contextual changes, and the mutual influences between the two.

Simply, the study of diversity and context should be moved to the fore of scholarly concern. Such scholarship would have important implications for policies and programs pertinent to individual and family life.

DIVERSITY, POLICIES, AND PROGRAMS

If the diversity- and context-sensitive developmental research promoted by developmental contextualism positively impacts policies and the programs derived from them, then such interventions will be designed to fit the diverse characteristics of the people served by, or involved in, these actions. Such diversity may pertain to variation in (a) family structure and function; and/or (b) developmental differences in the generations comprising a family.

As illustrated in Table 1.1 and in our discussion of the scholarship of Hernandez (1993), there is great historical and contemporary diversity in families and in the characteristics of the people who comprise them. People differ in their age; generational group (e.g., they may be young children, adult parents, or grandparents); race (i.e., their membership in a culturally defined group that is purported to share biological/reproductive characteristics); ethnicity (i.e., their membership in a culturally defined group that is purported to share historical and cultural characteristics, including in some cases geographical areas of group origin); physical attributes (e.g., their gender and possession of a physical disability); health status (e.g., the presence of an acute or chronic disease); sexual orientations (heterosexual, gay, lesbian, or bisexual); religions; and numerous psychological characteristics (e.g., their political affiliations, attitudes and values, and gender role and life style preferences).

The families within which such diverse people live are even more varied, as two or more individuals whose individual diversity *across* domains of characteristics, such as those noted above, combine to constitute a family unit. For instance, an intact family with children, comprised of a Latino and an Asian American adult, and a biological child with a chronic illness, differs from a single-parent family headed by a European American mother with two healthy children. In turn, a family involving a Latino parent of Puerto Rican ethnic background is different than one having a parent of Mexican ethnicity. These families could also involve a gay or a lesbian couple and their biological or adopted children, and such addition of variation would complicate further issues for policy development.

Listing the literally thousands, if not millions, of instances of family diversity that assuredly exist currently in our nation is certainly beyond the scope of this volume. Indeed, Wilson (1995; Wilson, Philip, Kohn, & Curry-El, 1995) has found that even *within* one demographic category of families—single-parent, female head-of-household families—there were as many as 18 different constellations of family types, for example, families wherein a biological father played a role in the family although he did not reside with the mother, families wherein a male who was not the non-biological father of the children was available to the family for some periods of time on a fairly regular basis, and families wherein other relatives (e.g., grandparents, aunts, or cousins) helped provide social support to the mother and her children. Similarly, Burton (1990) has found that in the families formed by African American teenage mothers there are several different types of family constellations that are present. For instance, there are families where the grandmother of the teenage mother's child (or children) takes on child rearing responsibilities and, at the other extreme, there are families where the oldest female child of the teenage mother has the responsibility for the rearing of her younger siblings.

The presence of such differences in the constitution of the family underscores the importance of the need to develop policies that recognize and address family diversity. At times, such policy innovations can involve nothing more than the relatively simple decision to allow people who are identifying themselves on government forms (e.g., in the Census) to specify in their own terms the racial and/or ethnic group with which they associate themselves.

At other times, however, the issues for policy development are much more complex—a point that should be obvious given the different domains of diversity we have just discussed. For instance, can we appropriately frame a "family" policy in the United States without recognizing that families with children differ from those without young people in them? And does not this issue get more complicated when we consider the fact that a family in which the children are very young is different from one with adolescent or grown children, and also different from one wherein the parents are themselves adult children having the responsibility of caring for their own aged parents? Should accommodations in family policy be made to recognize the great frequency in the United States of family dissolution and reconstitution (divorce and remarriage)? Should we develop policies that treat single-parent families formed when a teenage girl becomes an unmarried mother as different than single-parent families that are formed when a middle-aged woman with growing children is divorced or is widowed? Shall we develop policies that provide the same loan and health benefits to families involving gay and lesbian partners as we do to families involving heterosexual partners? And, in recognition of the trends about maternal employment, and thus of changing gender roles in America, should we develop policies to support specifically what is now a majority of women who seek to have families *and* careers outside of their homes?

In short, then, in the formulation of family policy there is abundant reason to consider all the ways in which groups may differ. However, is such a focus the only idea to derive from a consideration of human diversity? Moreover, is such a focus always possible, feasible, or even appropriate? We believe that there are more subtle implications of individual and family diversity for the development of family policy.

FAMILY DIVERSITY AND FAMILY POLICY: THE "DOUBLE-EDGED SWORD" OF DIFFERENTIATION AND GENERALIZATION

The diversity of the American family, and of the children, youth, and adults that comprise these institutions, means that any one family policy will not address adequately the individuality of the people to which it is directed (i.e., "one size fits all" does not work for pubic policy). Nevertheless, as political leaders accept the need to develop public policies that are more sensitive to this diversity, they also will be faced with the practical obstacles of cost and management that would be involved if they were to attempt to develop initiatives that were as diverse as the populations intended to be served by these actions. Accordingly, a much more subtle issue is involved in developing policies that are diversity sensitive, one captured perhaps by the question, "How much diversity matters in regard to a particular policy issue?"

For example, in developing a welfare-to-work strategy for single mothers, are the ethnic/racial differences between low-income, adolescent African American women, Latina women, and European American women necessary to consider? In turn, can all Latino adolescents be functionally treated in the same way or, in order to forge effective policies, will it be necessary to develop actions that are sensitive to the historical and cultural differences between Latinos of, for example, Mexican, Puerto Rican, and Caribbean heritage? In recognizing that "one size does not fit all" with regard to family policy, policy makers are nevertheless faced with a dilemma of deciding just what instances or degrees of diversity are necessary to consider, and which may be ignored, to design or implement particular policies for particular groups.

While we need to develop policies sensitive to diversity, then, we must be certain that different groups vary significantly in regard to policy-relevant dimensions. For instance, we cannot assume that just because people have different skin colors they therefore also vary in those characteristics that are pertinent to particular policy concerns. For example, in attempts to develop policies and programs aimed at enhancing the lives of African American and Latino families, do we need to formulate different welfare-to-work policies (for instance, involving support for home-based child care while mothers are receiving job training or more general education; cf. Kossek, Huber-Yoder, Castellino, & Lerner, 1997)? In addition to their ethnic/racial differences, do the two groups have enduring ethnic/cultural differences in regard to caregiving support provided by extended family members that would require different policies in regard to developing effective welfare-to-work programs?

Whereas there may be wide-spread beliefs or even stereotypes, about the ethnic/cultural differences between these two (and other) groups, the scholarship of McAdoo (1981, 1998b, 1999) provides facts that contradict such views. For instance, McAdoo (1999) notes that:

> When one analyzes these groups for commonalities, one finds strong similarities. There are very similar family patterns in

groups of color—Native American, Mexican American, African American, and Asian families. These are the common cultural patterns that have contributed to the resiliency of families of color. There are supportive social networks, flexible relationships within the family units, a strong sense of religiosity, extensive use of extended family helping arrangements, the adoption of fictive kin who become as family, and strong identification with their racial group. . . . The extended families of African Americans is practically the same as "familism" in Mexican Americans, but they are often never discussed together or compared. The respect that is given the elderly in Asian families is similar to the central roles of the elderly in Native American families. All of these groups have culturally evolved in unique ways that reflect the country of origin, the culture, and the geographic location of their groups, yet are very similar in their family patterns. (p. 210)

Accordingly, McAdoo's scholarship points to the "double-edged sword" of addressing the linkage between family diversity and family policy. On the one hand, we must be sensitive to the potentially distinctive characteristics of a particular racial or ethnic group, both to understand adequately that group and to design effective policies that derive from that understanding. On the other hand, we cannot ignore the commonalities that exist across diverse groups—commonalities which allow the formulation of general principles of family functioning and afford the creation of economies of scale in regard to the creation of policies and programs. Moreover, by allowing the articulation of the double-edged nature of the linkage between family diversity and family policy, McAdoo's ideas point more generally to the need to adopt a more nuanced conception of diversity.

For instance, McAdoo argues (McAdoo, 1998b) that family diversity is not just a between-group phenomenon but, as well, a within-group dimension. To illustrate, not only may distinct racial/ethnic groups possess cross-group commonalities as well as significant differences but, in addition, it may be that important variation exists within any racial/ethnic group. Indeed, it is possible that such intragroup variation may be more important in the development of policy than is intergroup variation.

As a consequence, then, in studying any dimension of family diversity (e.g., racial/ethnic variation, the presence of a handicapped parent or child, the occurrence of family violence or abuse, single-parent families, or socioeconomic differences) in relation to family policy, McAdoo's scholarship leads to: 1. an awareness of the need to be precise about why a particular dimension of family diversity is pertinent to a given policy issue; 2. sensitivity to the differences that exist between groups in regard to a relevant dimension of diversity; and 3. a recognition of the need to be sensitive to the potential significance of within-group variation. We may illustrate the significance of this tripartite perspective by a discussion of ethnic differences and, in turn, of the literature pertinent to the African American family.

THE ROLE OF ETHNIC VARIATION IN FAMILY DIVERSITY

The conception in America of family ethnic diversity has evolved over the last quarter century. For example, Mindel, Habenstein, and Roosevelt (1998), writing in the preface to the fourth edition of their edited text on ethnic families in America, note that:

> At the time of the publication of the first edition in the 1970s, the prevailing view of ethnicity seemed to be that the United States was an assemblage of mostly European ethnic groups who had been forged into new amalgam by means of a great "melting pot." Assimilation as a cultural value, the view that immigrants to this land should somehow give up their strange cultural ways, beliefs, and languages and adopt the "American" way, was dominant. The idea that separate ethnic group identification in the United States was valuable in its own right was only beginning to be appreciated. Competing notions of ethnic pride and ethnic self-determination which challenged the value of assimilation were in their infancy. (p. vii)

In support of Mindel, et al.'s (1988) contention about the pressures put on diverse immigrant groups to assimilate dominated American society until the last quarter-century, scholars such as Jacobson (1998; see, too, Brodkin, 1998; Ignatiev, 1995; Itzkovitz, 1998) discuss how, across this century up through World War II and the immediate post-war years, various groups (e.g., Jews) came to the United States in the context of federal laws that permitted virtually free immigration (through 1924) but in the face of attitudes (e.g., anti-Semitism) that cast the groups as distinct and non-White racial groups. In his book, *Whiteness of a different color: European immigrants and the alchemy of race,* Jacobson (1998) argues that Jews and other immigrant groups came to America and were categorized as not belonging to a race equivalent to European-Americans of Anglo-Saxon heritage. However, through their personal efforts to assimilate, their adoption of popular culture, their settling in areas (e.g., the suburbs) that enabled them to blend into the larger, "Anglo-Saxon" culture, and the presence of facilitative public policies (e.g., the GI Bill enacted after World War II), Jews and other immigrant groups (e.g., the Irish) became "White," that is, they became part of the predominant, European-American "race," exemplified by the "old" Anglo-Saxon "stock" (Brodkin, 1998; Heller, 1999; Ignatiev, 1995; Itzkovitz, 1998; Jacobson, 1998).

Of course, because of their skin color, such merging into the mainstream White "racial" culture was not feasible for most African Americans. Thus, through the time of the first edition of their book, Mindel, et al. (1998) saw a nation wherein ethnic diversity was an issue to be overcome by diverse individuals. Immigrants sought to transcend their identity or their categorization as a separate racial or ethnic group, attempting to become part of White American mainstream society. When this was not prototypically possible, as in the case of African Americans, a sense of being "The Other" (Brodkin, 1998) may have been an all-too-frequent result, one that could be associated with alienation and anger among members of the group—as well as with being the target of suspicion by and discrimination from the majority group. Another reaction might be a campaign for social justice, for societal equity.

It was in such a milieu of societal controversy involving the status in America of diverse racial and ethnic groups, that the first edition (in 1970) of the Mindel, et al., book appeared. Commenting on this period, they note that:

> the black civil rights struggle was not a somewhat forgotten memory, and "affirmative action" was still an emerging idea, its political repercussions not yet apparent. The political machines of big northern cities remained still largely under the control of representatives of European ethnic groups. (Mindel, et al., 1998, p. 1)

Mindel, et al. (1998) speculate that the alteration of views regarding ethnicity after the time that their book first appeared was due to the civil rights movements of the 1960s, the Vietnam War, and the American civil unrest associated with it during the 1960s and 1970s, and the new immigration laws which took effect in the 1960s. In regard to this latter potential influence, Mindel, et al. (1998, p. vii) observe that:

> The United States had been largely closed to new immigration after 1924, when a discriminatory law effectively barred immigrants from eastern and southern Europe and Asia. Beginning with the Immigration and Nationality Act of 1965, and later with the opening of the immigration doors to Cuban, Vietnamese, Soviet, and Salvadoran refugees, among others, as well as swelling numbers of immigrants who arrived and stayed on illegally, the nature of ethnicity in the United States changes profoundly.

Thus, Mindel, et al. (1998) underscore the intimate interplay among policy changes, broader contextual changes (for instance involving non-normative historical events such as wars, civil unrest, and illegal immigration) and, as such, the very conception of ethnic diversity that justifies the theoretical frame we propose for discussing the linkages between family diversity and family policy. Indeed, Mindel, et al. (1998) underscore the dynamic and thus relatively plastic nature of these linkages by reminding their readers that the "story" of ethnicity in America is still being told. They emphasize that:

> Currently the mood in the country, as reflected in recent changes in the immigration laws and the reduction of benefits to illegal immigrants, is on one of those anti-immigrant downturns that has afflicted this country almost from its inception" (p. viii). . . . The impact of the post-1965 waves of immigration with their increasing numbers, shifting national origins, and often illegal status has been unsettling for many individuals in older American groups. This sea of new faces is often seen as containing the seeds

of new serious social problems for American society or an acceleration of its ongoing breakdown. Talk show commentators and others express fears that the United States has lost control of its borders, its language, its "American" core values, and, increasingly, its ability to afford the cost of caring for new immigrants. (pp. 1-2)

Such reactions to diversity, to the extent they are influential at the historical period during which both Mindel, et al. (1998) and the present authors are writing, would create a political context for the development of family policies that may be argued to contrast significantly from the one that existed during the time that the 1965 Immigration and Nationality Act was being debated, enacted, and signed into law.

Of course, families differ in many dimensions. However, ethnicity is a major—indeed perhaps an organizing—one (e.g., Fisher, et al., 1998; Geertz, 1963; McAdoo, 1998b; Mindel, et al., 1998). An ethnic group "consists of those who share a unique social and cultural heritage that is passed on from generation to generation" (Mindel, et al., 1998, p. 6). This shared heritage has a powerful, cohesive influence on people identifying with it. According to Geertz (1963, p. 109):

> These congruities of blood, speech, custom, and so on, are seen to have an ineffable, at time overpowering, coerciveness in and of themselves. One is bound to one's kinsman, one's neighbor, one's fellow believer, *ipso facto*, as a result not merely of ones personal affection, practical necessity, common interest, or incurred obligation, but at least in great part by the virtue of some unaccountable absolute import attributed to the very tie itself. The general strength of such primordial bonds, and the types of them that are important, differ from person to person, from society to society, and from time to time. But for virtually every person, in every society, at almost all times, some attachments seem to flow from a sense of natural—some would say spiritual—affinity than from social interaction.

Thus, although ethnic ties may exist among people who are members of groups as general as European Americans, African Americans, Latinos, or Asian Americans, the integrative bonds described by Geertz (1963) may be organized on more subtle dimensions linked, for instance, to the particular country from which one's ancestors came, shared language or speech patterns, or historical experiences and religious traditions. Accordingly, senses of ethnicity and interpersonal affinity based on ethnic commonality may create as much variation within a particular broad grouping of people (e.g., European American or Latino) than between any two such groupings.

For example, in the Mindel, et al. (1998) volume the differences that exist among European American families from Irish, Greek, Italian, Polish, and Jewish families are discussed. Similarly, variation within Latino families is illustrated through discussions of groups from Mexican, Puerto Rican, and Cuban backgrounds. In turn, the diversity within Asian American families is illustrated by discussing groups whose heritage is Korean, Vietnamese, Chinese, Japanese, and Asian Indian. Given such within-group diversity, it would be a mistake to regard all people of, for instance, a common skin color as the same; it would be problematic to try to develop effective policies that ignored the ethnic differences that exist within as well as between groups. In this regard, McAdoo (1999, p. 208) has observed that "It is important to understand that the common element of being of color does not decide exactly what the life patterns of individuals will be."

ETHNIC DIVERSITY: THE "SAMPLE CASE" OF THE AFRICAN AMERICAN FAMILY

McAdoo (1998b) makes points—in regard to the diversity that exists with the African American community—that correspond to those forwarded by Mindel, et al. (1998b). Her discussion of African American families can elucidate, then, the double-edged character of the linkage between family diversity and family policy. She describes several features of the structure and function of African American families (e.g., the supportive role played by extended family members) that that are generalizable to the families of other racial/ethnic groups, at the same time explaining why African Americans cannot be seen as a monolithic group. She describes the rich within-group variation that exists with the African American population. For instance, she notes that:

> African-American families represent a range of different groups who have had diverse experiences. Given the many patterns of family life and socioeconomic levels in which African Americans have lived in North America, it is impossible to use median data to describe the situation today, yet authors almost consistently do so. Never has it been more obvious that the African American experience is not one reality. Some families have made major gains and are prospering; others are barely holding onto their gains; still others are sliding backward into economic distress. This socioeconomic diversity is increasing every day. Despite attempts by the media and academia to present African Americans as one social, and usually lower, class, it is important to understand that being of African descent does not in itself determine what the life pattern of an individual will be (McAdoo, 1998a). It has simply become more difficult for African Americans to excel in the present environment. . . . In the past, it has been suggested that African Americans could be divided into two groups, survivors and non-survivors, but this characterization was and continues to be too simplistic. We no longer can accurately describe the United States as two nations, one black and unequal and one white and equal. African-American families, in the main, do not fare as well as

Family Diversity and Family Policy 55

> families from groups who are not of color, but to explain African-American families only in relation to nonblack families would be a fallacy, for we would miss the essence and dynamics of African-American family life today. (McAdoo, 1998b, pp. 361-362)

The demographics and the structure and function of the African American family underscore McAdoo's points about the diversity that exists with the African American community. McAdoo (1998b, 1999) notes that by the year 2050 families of color will become the majority in North America. This change is being propelled by the fact that, since the 1980s, families of color are younger and larger than families not of color; the age and size characteristics of families of color that are associated with cultural orientations, and often, specifically, with religious beliefs about not limiting family size (McAdoo, 1998b, 1999). Thus, because of the age at which they begin having children and in relation to their beliefs about family size, families of color:

> will be in the age range of becoming parents far longer than most families. As a result, persons of color have more children per family, while nonethnic families have children at less than the replacement level. More children of color are being born, and few are born who are not of color. (McAdoo, 1999, p. 207)

Changes in the African American community exemplify these demographic trends. Between 1980 and 1990, the African American population increased by 26% and, by 1990, constituted about one-eighth, or 12.1%, of the overall American population (McAdoo, 1998b). By the year 2010, African Americans will be about one-seventh of the American population (McAdoo, 1998b). According to McAdoo (1998b, pp. 365-366), 53% of this population is female; about one-third of African Americans are under 18 years of age (the median age is 28 years); life expectancy is 69 years of age (with a higher expectancy for females, of 74 years, than for males, of 64 years); annual income is less than $25,000 for 62% and more than $50,000 for 12%; 63.1% have high school or higher degrees and 11.4% have college or higher degrees; and 43% of the 10 million African American householders own their own homes.

Structurally, African American families "tend to be multigenerational and to include different combinations of roles within the units" (McAdoo, 1998b, p. 368). This type of domestic arrangement of family units represents the "major distinction that can be made between families of African and European descent" (McAdoo, 1998b, p. 368). McAdoo explains the African American pattern as deriving from West Africa, wherein both partriarchical and matriarchal forms of the family have had traditions; however, all forms have involved a family unit of temporally stable adult relatives from multiple generations. Moreover, McAdoo notes that one component of extended family living arrangements is extensive helping systems that span families and households.

Such arrangements, embedded within multigenerational living, allows one to distinguish between family stability and marital stability (McAdoo, 1998b). The former type of stability is high in African American families, existing in one-parent, grand-parent, or two-parent households. It often involves a woman, her children, and another adult (e.g., a sister or grandparent), and constitutes a source of stable love and resources for children and a context that may be as supportive of the youth as is a two-parent one (McAdoo, 1998b). For instance, McAdoo (1981) found that, in a sample of 178 middle-income African American families involving 305 parents, the extended family help network was an important source of support. Both kin and fictive kin were found to provide this support, both to families who had recently become socioeconomically mobile (and moved into the middle-income level) and to families who had experienced one or two generations of middle-income status. Indicative of the acceptance and utility of this extended family support system, the families studied by McAdoo (1981) reported that they did not feel that the obligations that existed for reciprocity for received help were excessive.

In contrast to the system that maintains family stability, McAdoo (1998b) notes that marriage is not a modal life style choice for African Americans. More so than for the American population in general, African Americans are not only postponing marriage but are deciding not to marry at all. For instance, McAdoo (1998b) indicates that in 1991 only 44% of African American adults were married (compared with 64% in 1970), and that the divorce rate for African American women is twice as high as it is for European American women.

Perhaps as a consequence of these marital patterns, there is only a 20% chance that African American children will live in two-parent families through the age of 16 years (McAdoo, 1998b). Indeed, McAdoo notes that only 5% of African American children (as compared to 20% of European-American children) live in homes where there is a father who acts in the breadwinner role and a mother who acts in the homemaker roles (i.e., the roles that Hernandez, 1993, has described as prototypic of the "Ozzie and Harriet" family). Indeed, whereas more than one-third (i.e., 37%) of African American children live with both parents almost half (i.e., 49.3%) live with their mothers but not their fathers (whereas only 5.4% lives with their father but not their mothers) (McAdoo, 1998b, p. 372).

Independent of their living arrangements, however, McAdoo emphasizes that African American children are imbued strongly with positive values about self, others, and community. She notes that:

> Parents of young children have been found to value self-sufficiency, a strong work orientation, positive racial attitudes, perseverance, and respect for the mother's role in the family (McAdoo & Crawford, 1991). These values have been found to be highly regarded by single mothers (McAdoo, 1991a). There is often a strong blend of the spirit of volunteerism and service to others who may be less fortunate. Family-oriented values and values that reinforce African American culture have been found in the history and oral traditions of many grandparents, and, most important, these histories and traditions are passed down from one generation to another. (McAdoo, 1998b, p. 375)

The inculcation of these values have been reinforced by the African American church, which McAdoo (1998b) identifies as one of the special strengths of African American families. However, despite the commonality of values that may be imbued in children through their families' involvement in the church, McAdoo (1998b) stresses that there is also great diversity among African Americans in the types of churches with which they are affiliated. African Americans are members of the Protestant, Catholic, and Moslem religions and, as well, "an ever-growing number of African Americans belong to other 'nontraditional' religious organizations" (McAdoo, 1998b, p. 376).

CONCLUSIONS

Understanding family diversity and using such knowledge for the formulation of public policy requires a multidimensional understanding of diversity. As exemplified by the scholarship of McAdoo (e.g., 1981, 1991, 1998a, 1998b, 1999; McAdoo & Crawford, 1991) one must be sensitive to *both* the features of family structure and function that *vary* across racial/ethnic (or other types of individual difference attributes of) groups and those features that are *common* across groups.

In addition, however, one must be aware that a racial/ethnic group is not an undifferentiated entity. There is within-group variation. Dimensions of diversity other than race/ethnicity (e.g., religion, socioeconomic status, vocational or professional affiliations, physical ability status, and political values) exist within any group and, for particular issues, these within-group differences may be more important for the formulation of diversity-sensitive policies than are between-group differences. For instance, in discussions of whether public funding should be made available for abortions, the key dimensions of diversity may not be racial/ethnic ones but, instead, affiliations with particular political parties or religious denominations.

In sum, then, in developing diversity-sensitive family policies at least three questions must be addressed. In what ways are particular family groups different? In what ways are particular family groups similar? And what are the dimensions of diversity that exist within a particular family group?

Family Diversity and the Formulation of Family Policy

Within the confines of one book it is not possible to address the above three questions for each instance of the vast array of diverse families that exist. What we can do, however, is provide examples of how the theoretical frame we bring to the study of such questions can help address the complexities of aligning policy with the diversity of individuals comprising America's families. That is, to illustrate the importance of contextual and developmental diversity for policies pertinent to both families and individuals, it is useful to provide three sample cases of the application of developmental contextual thinking to policy.

A first example derives from the attention within developmental contextualism to the historical embeddedness of family structure and function. Today, the challenges of parenting youth, and particularly adolescents, are complicated by both the diversity of family structures that characterizes the American family (see the discussion in Chapter 1 of the work of Hernandez, 1993, and Lerner, et al., 1995) *and* the historically unprecedented incidence of comorbid risk behaviors present within the adolescents population (e.g., Dryfoos, 1990; Hamburg, 1992; Lerner, 1995). For instance, some scholars have estimated that about 50% of the approximately 35.5 million American youth between the ages of 10 and 19 years (Yax, 1998) engage in two or more of the major types of high risk behaviors (i.e., drug and alcohol use; delinquency; school failure; and unsafe sex). In fact, adolescents' engagement in unsafe sexual practices has been associated with many other serious behavioral and health problems, including sexually transmitted diseases, teenage pregnancy, and teenage parenting (Carnegie Corporation of New York, 1995; Dryfoos, 1990; Hamburg, 1992). For instance, every minute of the day in America an adolescent gives birth (Children's Defense Fund, 1996). As a consequence, the difficulties of parenting contemporary American adolescents is complicated by the fact that many adolescents are themselves parents. Accordingly, a generationally differentiated approach to policies is needed (Smith, 1995, 1997; Smith, Blank, & Collins, 1992; Smith, Fairchild, & Groginsky, 1997; Smith & Zaslow, 1995; Zaslow, Tout, Smith, & Moore, 1998) to address adequately the historically unprecedented challenges of parenting adolescents when, at the same time, many of them may also be parents.

Our first sample case, then, will discuss this dual challenge of parenting adolescents and adolescents as parents. The import of this challenge is that a multigenerational perspective about family policy must be pursued while, at the same time, paying particular attention to the historically unprecedented problems created by the incidence of teenage parenting and its co-occurrence with other risk behaviors. These implications for policy lead to the other two sample cases we present.

In our second sample case we focus on welfare and welfare reform. We discuss the literature pertinent to these foci (e.g., Blum, 1992; Bogenschneider, 1994, 1997; Bogenschneider, & Corbett, 1995, 1997; Bogenschneider, Corbett, & Bell, 1997; Bogenschneider, Corbett, Bell, & Linney, 1997; Bogenschneider, Ragsdale, & Linney, 1995; Lerner, Castellino, et al., 1995; Smith, 1995, 1997; Smith, et al., 1992; Smith, et al., 1997; Smith & Zaslow, 1995; Zaslow, et al., 1998) and emphasize that policy must be developed in a manner that supports directly the positive development of both the parent and child generations present in welfare families. In the past, welfare policies have been directed typically to the mother, based on the assumption that by taking steps to enhancing her financial situation benefits to the child would accrue. As a consequence of such thinking, Aid to Families with Dependent Children (AFDC) was often the de facto "child policy" in the United States (Hahn, 1994). In other words, there was no explicit policy in the United States for the positive development of its children. There is still none today. Accordingly, the final sample case we offer is associated with the need for a national youth policy (Benson, 1997; Damon, 1997; Lerner, 1995; McAdoo, 1998b, 1999; Pittman & Irby, 1996).

5 THE PARENTING OF ADOLESCENTS AND ADOLESCENTS AS PARENTS

Parenting is both a biological and a social process (Lerner, Castellino, et al., 1995; Tobach & Schneirla, 1968). It is the term summarizing the set of behaviors involved across life in the relations among organisms who are usually conspecifics, and typically members of different generations or, at the least, of different birth cohorts. Parenting interactions provide resources across the generational groups and function in regard to domains of survival, reproduction, nurturance, and socialization.

Thus, parenting is a complex process, involving much more than a mother or father providing food, safety, and succor to an infant or child. Parenting involves bidirectional relationships between members of two (or more) generations; can extend through all or major parts of the respective life spans of these groups; may engage all institutions within a culture (including educational, economic, political, and social ones); and is embedded in the history of a people—as that history occurs within the natural and designed settings within which the group lives (Ford & Lerner, 1992). Given, then, the temporal variation that constitutes history, the variation of culture and its institutions that exist in different physical and designed ecological niches, and the variation—within and across generations—in strategies for and behaviors designed to fit with these niches, we may note that *diversity* is a key substantive feature of parenting behavior. Focus on this variation, rather than on central tendencies, is necessary in order to understand parenting adequately. In addition, since there are multiple levels of organization that change interdependently over both ontogenetic and historical time (Lerner & Lerner, 1989; Tobach & Greenberg, 1984), *context*, as well as diversity, is an important feature of parenting.

As we emphasized in Chapter 3, developmental contextualism is a theory of human development (Lerner, 1986, 1991, 1992; Lerner, Castellino, et al., 1995) that focuses on the changing *relations*—or, better, coactions (Gottlieb, 1997)—between the developing individual, and his or her context. We believe developmental contextualism is a perspective that is useful for understanding the contemporary challenges involved in studying adolescents and parenting *and* for designing programs pertinent to promoting the positive development of youth—in relation to enhancing the parenting they receive and/or to addressing the challenges faced by adolescents who are in the role of parents. That is, the challenges of adolescence derive from the fact that youth today are both in need of parenting that promotes their positive development and, *at the same time*, historically unprecedented numbers of adolescents are themselves becoming parents and, typically, unmarried parents (Children's Defense Fund, 1996).

Although we shall return again to the implications of developmental contextualism for the design of youth policies and programs, we should reiterate here the point that the contemporary context within which we may study the intersection of the life stage of adolescence and the role of parenting is characterized by an historically unprecedented coincidence of the need to understand both (a) how to parent adolescents; *and* (b) adolescents *as* parents. We discuss each of these topics successively.

PARENTING: CHILD REARING STYLES, SOCIALIZATION, AND PARENT-ADOLESCENT RELATIONSHIPS

The key function of a child's family is to raise the young person in as healthy a manner as possible (e.g., see Bornstein, 1995). The parents' role is to provide the child with a safe, secure, nurturant, loving, and supportive environment that allows the offspring to have a happy and healthy youth. This sort of experience allows the youth to develop the knowledge, values, attitudes, and behaviors necessary to become an adult making a productive contribution to self, family, community, and society (Lerner, Castellino, et al., 1995).

What a parent does to fulfill these "duties" of his or her role is termed *parenting*. In other words, parenting is a term that summarizes behaviors used by a person—usually, but, of course, not exclusively, the mother or father—to raise a child. Given the above-described characteristics of this set of activities, it is clear that parenting is the major function of the family.

We noted earlier (see Table 1.1), that adolescents live in different family structures. This variation influences both the way parents interact with youth and, in turn, the behavior of adolescents. For instance, in a study of urban African American adolescents living in either (1) single-mother, (2) stepparent, (3) dual parent, (4) mother-with-extended-family (e.g., grandparent, aunt, or uncle), or (5) extended-family-only settings (e.g., only an aunt is present), the social support provided to youth was generally the same across family types, with one exception: Youth living in single-mother families were given *more* support than the youth in the other four family types (Zimmerman, Salem, & Maton, 1995).

In turn, support to mothers, especially when provided by relatives, can enhance adolescent and maternal adjustment, and improve the mother's parenting skills (Taylor & Roberts, 1995). For example, among 14- to 19-year-old African American youth, social support from kin was related to self-reliance and good school grades. However, when kinship support was low the youth experienced feelings of distress (Taylor, 1996). Although differences in academic achievement and high school grades are slight among youth living in either intact, single-parent, and remarried families, large differences exist with regard to school drop-out (Zimiles & Lee, 1991). Students from intact families are *least* likely to drop out. Similarly, youth from such families are less likely to experiment with drugs than are adolescents from single-parent families (Turner, Irwin, & Millstein, 1991).

Of course, adults differ in the ways in which they enact their role as parents, showing different styles of raising children. Differences in child rearing styles are associated with important variation in adolescent development.

CHILD REARING STYLES IN ADOLESCENCE

The classic research of Diana Baumrind (1967, 1971) resulted in the identification of three major types of child rearing styles: authoritative, authoritarian, and permissive. The first style of rearing is marked by parental warmth, the use of rules and reasoning (induction) to promote obedience and keep discipline, non-punitive punishment (e.g., using "time out" or "grounding" instead of physical punishment), and consistency between statements and actions, and across time (Baumrind, 1971; Lamborn, Mounts, Steinberg, & Dornbusch, 1991). Authoritarian parents are not warm, stress rigid adherence to the rules they set (obey just because the parents are setting the rules), emphasize the power of their role, and use physical punishment for transgressions (Baumrind, 1971; Belsky, Lerner, & Spanier, 1984). Permissive parents do not show consistency in their use of rules, may have a "laissez-faire" attitude towards their child's behaviors (i.e., they may either not attend to the child, or let him or her do whatever he or she wants), and may give the child anything he or she requests; their style may be characterized as being either more of a peer or, instead, as an independent "observer" of their child. Indeed, because of the diversity of behavioral patterns that can characterize the permissive parenting style, Maccoby and Martin (1983) proposed that this approach to parenting can best be thought of as two distinct types: indulgent (e.g., "If my child wants something, I give it to her") and neglectful (e.g., "I really don't know what my child is up to. I don't really keep close tabs on her").

Whether the three categories of rearing style originally proposed by Baumrind (1967, 1971), the four categories suggested by Maccoby and Martin (1983), or other labels are used, it is clear that the behavioral variation summarized by use of the different categories is associated with differences in adolescent behavior and development (Lamborn, et al., 1991). For example, in a study of over 4,000 14- to 18-year-olds, adolescents with authoritative parents had more social competence and fewer psychological and behavioral problems than youth with authoritarian, indulgent, or neglectful parents (Lamborn, et al., 1991). In fact, youth with neglectful parents were the least socially competent and had the most psychological and behavioral problems of any group of adolescents in the study. In turn, youth with authoritarian parents were obedient and conformed well to authority, but had poorer self-concepts than other adolescents. Finally, while youth with indulgent parents had high self-confidence, they more often abused substances, and misbehaved and were less engaged in school.

Similarly, in a study of about 10,000 high school students, adolescents whose parents are accepting, firm, and democratic achieve higher school grades, are more self-reliant, less anxious and depressed, and less likely to engage in delinquent behavior than are youth with parents using other rearing styles (Steinberg, Mounts, Lamborn, & Dornbusch, 1991). This influence of authoritative parenting held for youth of different ethnic and socioeconomic backgrounds and regardless of whether the adolescent's family was intact. Moreover, adolescents with authoritative parents are more likely to have well-rounded peer groups that admire both adult as well as youth values and norms (e.g., academic achievement/school success and athletics/social popularity, respectively; Durbin, Darling, Steinberg, & Brown, 1993). In turn, youth with uninvolved parents had peer groups that did not support adult norms or values, and boys with indulgent parents were in peer groups that stressed fun and partying (Durbin, et al., 1993).

Considerable additional research confirms the generally positive influence on adolescent development of authoritative parenting and, in turn, of the developmental problems that emerge in youth when parents are authoritarian, permissive, indulgent, or uninvolved (e.g., Almeida & Galambos, 1991; Baumrind, 1991; Brown, Mounts, Lamborn, & Steinberg, 1993; Feldman & Wood, 1994; Melby & Conger, 1996; Paulson, 1994; Simons, Johnson, & Conger, 1994; Wentzel, Feldman, & Weinberger, 1991). Moreover, this research confirms as well that the positive influences of authoritative parenting extend to the adolescent's choice of, or involvement with, peers (e.g., Brown, et al., 1993). Thus, the influence of parents is often highly consistent with the influence of peers among adolescents (Lerner & Galambos, 1998).

SOCIALIZATION IN ADOLESCENCE

Whichever style parents use to rear their adolescents, the goal of parenting is to raise a child who is healthy and successful in life, can contribute to self and to society, and accepts and works to further the social order. The process—the behaviors that are used over time—to reach these goals is termed *socialization*. Although all societies socialize their youth (in order that, as future contributors to society, they can contribute to society's survival and prosperity), there are marked differences in what different societies, or groups within a society, want to see in a youth that has been "successfully" socialized. Said another way, there is great diversity in the specific goals parents have in socializing their youth.

One way of illustrating this contextual variation and, as well, of judging whether parents and society at large have been successful in shaping youth to accept social values, is to ask youth what it means to be a good or a bad child. In one study that took this approach, American, Japanese, and Chinese adolescents were asked, "What is a bad kid?" (Crystal & Stevenson, 1995). In America, youth answered that a lack of self-control and substance abuse were the marks of being bad. In China, a youth who engaged in acts against society was judged as bad. In Japan, a youth who created disruptions of interpersonal harmony was regarded as bad.

Another way of understanding the socialization process is to see how immigrants to a new country give up the values and customs of their country of origin and adopt those of their new one—a set of changes termed *acculturation*. This approach was used in a series of studies involving youth of Chinese ancestry, who were either first generation Americans (their parents were born in China and immigrated before the adolescent was born) or second generation Americans (their grandparents were born in China, but their parents had been born in the United States). These youth were contrasted to Chinese adolescents from Hong Kong, youth of Chinese ancestry whose parents had immigrated to Australia, European American youth, and Anglo Australian youth. In one study, both first and second generation Chinese American youth were similar to the non-immigrant youth groups in their levels of adolescent problems (Chiu, Feldman, & Rosenthal, 1992). However, immigration resulted in lowered perceptions of parental control, but it was not related to views about their parents' warmth. In turn, Chinese American adolescents' value on the family as a residential unit changed across the generations (in the direction of placing less value on the family for this function). This variation was consistent in direction with acculturation to both Anglo Australian and European American values (Feldman, Mont-Reynaud, & Rosenthal, 1992). However, with regard to mean levels, the Chinese Americans still differed from these other groups in this value.

Still another approach to understanding socialization is to appraise whether different groups within a society direct their youth to comparable developmental achievements. Research in Israel, for instance, suggests that youth from Arab Israeli families are raised to view the father as having more power than the mother. In turn, Jewish Israeli youth see more maternal than paternal power (Weller, Florian, & Mikulincer, 1995). Similarly, in Japan, problems of adolescent adjustment are most likely to occur for boys who are aligned with their mothers, but whose mothers and fathers disagree about socialization practices (Gjerde & Shimizu, 1995). In turn, male and female adolescent immigrants from Third World countries to Norway differ in their attitudes toward acculturation (Sam, 1995). Although both groups place a lot of importance on maintaining their cultural heritage, boys favor acculturation more than girls.

In the United States, while there is evidence of consistency in some socialization practices across diverse groups (e.g., with regard to the development of mental health among Latino and European American youth; Knight, Virden, & Roosa, 1994), there is also research indicating that practices differ in different American groups. For instance, African American parents more frequently discuss prejudice with their adolescent children than do Japanese American or Mexican American parents (Phinney & Chavira, 1995). In addition, both African American and Japanese American parents emphasize adaptation to society more so than do Mexican American parents.

How successful are parents' attempts at socialization? By virtue of the fact that society continues to evolve and is not characterized by intergenerational warfare or revolution, and that the vast majority of youth become contributing adults to society, we can conclude that socialization "works," that the "apple does not fall far from the tree" (Adelson, 1970; Lerner, 1986). Indeed, during adolescence very few families—estimates are between 5% to 10%—experience a major deterioration in the parent-child relationship (Steinberg et al, 1991). Moreover, not only do parents expect to see change in their sons' and daughters' behaviors as they socialize them during adolescence (Freedman-Doan, Arbreton, Harold, & Eccles, 1993), but— through their interactions on a day-to-day basis—parents can model and/or shape the cognitive, emotional and behavioral attributes they desire to see in their offspring (e.g., Eisenberg & McNally, 1993; Larson & Richards, 1994; Simons, et al., 1991; Whitbeck, 1987). It is through the relationships that parents and their adolescent children have that the most immediate bases are provided of youth behavior and development.

PARENT-CHILD RELATIONSHIPS IN ADOLESCENCE

There are a range of behaviors and associated emotions exchanged between parents and their adolescent offspring. Some of these exchanges involve positive and healthy behaviors and others involve the opposite. Some of the outcomes for adolescent development of these exchanges reflect good adjustment and individual and social success, whereas other outcomes reflect poor adjustment and problems of development. As is true for all facets of human development, there is diversity in the nature and implications of parent-child relations in adolescence.

Parent-adolescent relationships involving supportive behaviors and positive emotions

Among American youth, warm parental interactions are associated with effective problem solving ability in both the adolescent and the family as a whole. However, hostile interactions are associated with destructive adolescent problem solving behaviors (Ge, Best, Conger, & Simons, 1996; Rueter & Conger, 1995). Similarly, among German adolescents, parental behavior marked by approval and attention to the positive behavior of the youth is associated with an adolescent who feels he or she is capable of controlling events that can affect him or her (Krampen, 1989). However, when parental behaviors disparage the child and fail to attend to his or her specific behavior, the adolescent feels that chance determines what happens to him or her in life.

As illustrated by the above studies, warmth, nonhostility, and closeness seem to be characteristics of parent-adolescent interaction that are associated with positive outcomes among youth. Other research confirms these linkages. Feelings of closeness in the parent-adolescent relationship is related to parents' views of their parenting as satisfying to them, and to the youth's self-esteem and his or her participation in family activities (Paulson, Hill, & Holmbeck, 1991).

In turn, nonhostile parent-adolescent relations are associated with better adjustment by the adolescent to the transition to middle school and greater peer popularity (Bronstein, Fitzgerald, Briones, & Pieniadz, 1993). In addition, nonhostility is related to a better self-concept for girls and better classroom behavior for boys. Moreover, when parents are attuned to their child's development and support his or her autonomy in decision making, the youth is better adjusted and *gains* in self-esteem across the junior high school transition (Lord, Eccles, & McCarthy, 1994). Furthermore, parental religiosity, cohesive family relationships, and low interpersonal conflict are associated with low levels of problem behaviors and with self-regulation among rural African American youth (Brody, Stoneman, & Flor, 1996).

The characteristics of parent-child interaction that are associated with positive outcomes for the adolescent are similar in that they reflect support for, and acceptance of, the developing youth. Indeed, when parent-adolescent relationships provide support for the youth's behaviors, interest, and activities, numerous positive developmental outcomes are likely to occur. For instance, support has been associated with better school grades and scholastic self-concept (DuBois, Eitel, & Felner, 1994); perceiving that social relationships could be more beneficial to one's development than risky (East, 1989); being more satisfied with one's life (Young, Hiller, Norton, & Hill, 1995); and a decreased likelihood of involvement in drinking, delinquency, and other problem behaviors (Barnes & Farrell, 1992).

Certainly, receiving support from one's parents may elicit in the young person feelings of positive regard or emotions characterized by a sense of attachment. When such emotions occur in adolescence, positive outcomes for the youth are seen. For instance, parent-child relations marked by attachment are associated with high self-perceived competence, especially across the transition to junior high school, and with low feelings of depression or anxiety (Papini & Roggman, 1992). In addition, attachment is linked to feeling cohesive with one's family (Papini, Roggman, & Anderson, 1991). Other research also has found relationships among attachment, a positive sense of self, and low levels of problematic behaviors/emotions, such as depression (Kenny, Moilanen, Lomax, & Brabeck, 1993).

In sum, then, parent-child relationships marked by behaviors supportive of the youth and by positive feelings connecting the generations are associated with psychologically and socially healthy developmental outcomes for the adolescent. However, some families do not have parent-child relations marked by support and positive emotions, and no family has such exchanges all the time. Families experience conflict and negative emotions. Such exchanges also influence the adolescent but, as we might expect, the outcomes for youth of these influences differ from those associated with support and positive emotions.

Parent-adolescent relations involving conflict and stress

Family conflicts seem inevitable (Fisher & Johnson, 1990). At the least, conflicts are a ubiquitous part of all families at some times in their history. And the reasons for these conflicts vary. For example, adolescents report that conflicts often arise because they feel that parents are not providing the emotional support they want, or because youth or parents believe the other generation is not meeting the expectations held for them, or because of a lack of consensus about family or societal values (Fisher & Johnson, 1990).

In turn, in a study of over 1,800 Latino, African American, and European American parents of adolescents, conflicts were said to occur in the main over everyday matters, such as chores and style of dress, rather than with regard to substantive issues, such as sex and drugs (Barber, 1994). [Similar findings were reported in research conducted a generation earlier (Lerner & Knapp, 1975), suggesting that the nature of parents' views of reasons for arguing with their children may not change very much across time.] Parents from all racial/ethnic groups reported arguing about the same issues; however, European American parents reported more conflict than parents from the other two groups (Barber, 1994).

Moreover, although other research reports that adolescents and their parents are in conflict about the same sorts of issues—chores, appearance, and politeness—there is a decrease in arguments about these issues as the adolescent develops (Galambos & Almeida, 1992). However, conflict over finances tend to increase at older age levels. In turn, as youth develop, they are less likely to concede an argument to parents. As a result, conflicts may be left unresolved, especially, it seems, in families with boys (Smetana, Yau, & Hanson, 1991). The presence of conflicts between youth and parents is, then, a fact of family life during adolescents. Arguments with their youngsters are events with which parents must learn to cope.

Nevertheless, despite its developmental course, the presence of conflict at any point in the parent-adolescent relationship may influence the behavior and development of the youth. For instance, family conflicts may lead the adolescent to think negatively about himself or herself, and can even eventuate in his or her thinking about suicide (Shagle & Barber, 1993). In addition, conflict is associated with "externalizing" problems (e.g., such as hostility) among youth (Mason, et al., 1994). In adolescent girls, the experience of menarche and as a consequence less positive emotions and more negative ones characterize adolescent-parent exchanges (Holmbeck & Hill, 1991; Steinberg, 1987). In short, then, conflicts in the parent-adolescent relationship result in problems in youth development (Rubenstein & Feldman, 1993). A vicious cycle may be created in that, in turn, adolescent problems can increase parent-adolescent conflicts (Maggs & Galambos, 1993).

Moreover, the negative emotions exchanged between adolescents and their parents can themselves result in problems for the youth. For instance, fathers' feelings of stress are associated with adolescents' emotional and behavioral problems (Compas, 1989) and, as well, maternal stress is associated with "internalizing" problems (e.g., anxiety, depression) in adolescent boys and with poor school grades for adolescent girls.

The process through which parents' stress is linked to adolescent problems seems to involve the experience of depression in parents as a consequence of their stress which, in turn, disrupts effective parental discipline and leads to adolescent problem behaviors (Conger, Patterson, & Ge, 1995). Other research finds that parental depression is associated with depression in youth (Gallimore & Kurdek, 1992), and that ineffective parenting behaviors (e.g., low self-restraint among fathers) eventuates in problem behaviors in their offspring (Baumrind, 1991; D'Angelo, Weinberger, & Feldman, 1995; Feldman & Weinberger, 1994; Simons, et al., 1991).

Moreover, parents of tenth graders with conduct problems are more hostile than parents of tenth graders with depression (Ge, et al., 1996). In addition, parents of tenth graders who are *both* depressed and showing problem behaviors have high levels of hostility and low levels of warmth when their children are in Grades 7, 8, and 9. Similarly, depression among both European American and Asian American adolescents is associated with family relations marked by low warmth and acceptance and high levels of conflict with mothers and fathers (Greenberger & Chen, 1996). In addition, anger, hostility, coercion, and conflict shown by both parents and siblings have a detrimental effect on adolescent adjustment (Pike, et al., 1996).

Clearly, then, parents' negative emotions can lead, through the creation of problematic parenting behaviors, to negative outcomes in adolescent development. Moreover, the presence of problem behaviors in parents per se is linked to problems in adolescent development. For instance, psychiatric disorders among parents are related to the occurrence of antisocial and hostile behaviors among adolescents (Ge, et al., 1996). In addition, problem drinking or alcoholism in parents is associated with alcohol use and abuse problems in their adolescent offspring—a relation that occurs in European American, African American, and Latino families (Barrera, Li, & Chassin, 1995; Hunt, Streissguth, Kerr, & Olson, 1995; Peterson, Hawkins, Abbott, & Catalano, 1994). Similarly, parental drug use results in a host of behavioral, cognitive, and self-esteem problems in their offspring (Kandel, Rosenbaum, & Chen, 1994). Maternal smoking is associated with smoking in their adolescent children (Kandel & Wu, 1995) and, in fact, parental substance use in general is linked to numerous problems of adolescent personal and social behaviors, including experience with the substances (drugs, alcohol, cigarettes, etc.) used by parents (e.g., Andrews, Hops, Ary, & Tildesley, 1993; Stice & Barrera, 1995). Moreover, when fathers have an emotionally distant relationship with their wives and, as a consequence, turn to their adolescent daughters for intimacy and affection, the daughters show depression, anxiety, and low self-esteem (Jacobvitz & Bush, 1996).

In short, the rearing of adolescents is not accomplished in the same way and with the same outcomes by all parents. Adults vary in their parenting styles and the manner in which they socialize their children. This variation is linked to different individual characteristics of parents and, as well, to the features of the proximal and distal contexts within which parents and families are embedded. This variation is associated also with differences in other contextual factors—relating, for instance, to parental education, family social support, parental mental health, family stability, and poverty.

For instance, IQ scores for youth are lower in larger families, wherein the mother's educational attainment and the family's social support are low, and where the family is of minority background and poor (Sameroff, Seifer, Baldwin, & Baldwin, 1993; Taylor, 1996). In turn, in regard to family stability, there is a considerable body of research that indicates that divorce is associated with social, academic, and personal adjustment problems, including those associated with early initiation of sexual behavior (e. g., Brody & Forehand, 1990; Carson, Madison, & Santrock, 1987; Demo & Acock, 1988; Doherty & Needle, 1991; Hetherington, 1991; Hetherington, Cox, & Cox, 1985; Simons, et. al, 1994; Wallerstein, 1986; Whitbeck, Simons, & Kao, 1994; Zaslow, 1988, 1989). In addition, parent-child relations are less hierarchical and children are pushed to grow up faster in divorced families (Smetana, 1993).

The period following separation and divorce is quite stressful for youth (Doherty & Needle, 1991), especially if the adolescent is caught between divorced parents engaged in continuing, conflictual, and hostile interactions (Brody & Forehand,

1990; Buchanan, Maccoby, & Dornbusch, 1991). Furthermore, in some cases there are gender differences in the reaction of adolescents to divorce. For instance, although girls tend to react more negatively than boys prior to the parents' separation, they also tend to adapt better than boys after the divorce (Doherty & Needle, 1991; Hetherington, et al., 1985).

In the case of remarriage, there is evidence that although both male and female adolescents may have difficulty interacting with stepfathers, girls may have particular problems (Lee, Burkam, Zimiles, & Ladewski, 1994). Moreover, both male and female adolescents show no improvement in relationships with their stepfathers, or in behavior problems (e.g., regarding school grades) associated with the divorce—and this is the case even two years or more after the remarriage (Hetherington, 1991; Lee, et al., 1994).

In turn, living under the custody of one's natural father is linked as well to problems for both male and female adolescents (Lee, et al., 1994). For instance, adolescents living with their fathers adjust more poorly than youth living in other arrangements (e.g., with their mothers), a reaction that seems to be due to the closeness they have with, and the monitoring provided by, the parent with whom they are living (Buchanan, Maccoby, & Dornbusch, 1992). On the other hand, living with a stepfather, as compared to living with a stepmother, is associated with more positive self-esteem among both male and female adolescents (Fine & Kurdek, 1992).

Effects of maternal employment

After divorce, it is still the case that most youth live with their mothers, often for at least a period in a single-parent household (Furstenberg & Cherlin, 1991). Moreover, because of unwed pregnancies or paternal death, almost one-fourth of *all* American families are headed by a single female (Center for the Study of Social Policy, 1995). These women must support themselves and their children and thus, in such contexts, maternal employment is virtually a necessity.

Of course, women work outside the home even when they live in intact, two-parent families. Indeed, the majority of American mothers work outside the home, and do so for personal, social, and economic reasons that correspond to those found among men (Hernandez, 1993; J. Lerner, 1994).

Despite their reasons for working, maternal employment per se has generally not been found to have adverse affects on the personal or social development of youth (J. Lerner & Galambos, 1985, 1991). Adolescents whose mothers work outside the home do not differ from youth with non-employed mothers in regard to variables such as adjustment (Armistead, Wierson, & Forehand, 1990; Galambos & Maggs, 1990); the nature of the mother-adolescent relationship (Galambos & Maggs, 1990); adolescent responsibility and self-management (Keith, Nelson, Schlabach, & Thompson, 1990); and adolescent sexual attitudes and behaviors (Wright, Peterson, & Barnes, 1990).

Maternal employment can affect the mother's sense of "role strain," that is, the feeling that she is finding it difficult to balance the demands of her role of worker with the demands of her role as mother; or simply when she is dissatisfied with her

Family Diversity and Family Policy

role. Such role strain occurs when the mother feels there is a poor match between her aspirations or education and her job duties (Joebgen & Richards, 1990), or when she is in the midst of work transitions (Flanagan & Eccles, 1993). Simply, the mother feels stress because of the nature of her multiple roles. When such stress or role strain is experienced, an influence on adolescent adjustment can occur (Galambos, Sears, Almeida, & Kolaric, 1995; J. Lerner, 1994; J. Lerner & Galambos, 1985, 1991).

Parental work and adolescents in self-care

In addition, there may be implications for youth simply because, when their mother is at work, there is no parent in the home. Indeed, a mother's time at work is obviously associated with the amount of unsupervised time a youth experiences after, and sometimes before, school (Muller, 1995; Richards & Duckett, 1994). Unsupervised time, especially the hours of 3:00 p.m. to 8:00 p.m., represents a problem period for youth, who often do not spend their time profitably during such periods (i.e., they "just hang out"), or engage in high risk and/or illegal behaviors during such times (Carnegie Corporation of New York, 1992). However, in such cases it is the lack of supervision and not maternal employment per se that is the source of these difficulties for youth.

These problems can be counteracted. For example, when parents exert firm control over the way their youngsters spend time in "self-care" at home, problem behaviors can be reduced (Galambos & Maggs, 1991). In addition, effective community programs for youth, for example, 4-H, Boys and Girls Clubs, and community athletics, can provide youth with attractive, positive, and productive ways to spend their time. Current opinion among leaders of such youth-serving organizations is that if such community programs are strengthened, young adolescents will have richer experiences and fewer life problems (Carnegie Corporation of New York, 1992).

We will return to a fuller discussion of the characteristics of youth programs that appear to positively influence the development of adolescents. However, we should note that here the positive effect of community programs may not be as readily achievable when the parents in a family are themselves adolescents. In such cases, the risks to offspring are increased. "Adolescents as parents" represents the second scholarly focus we must address in order to understand the contemporary linkage between adolescence and parenting. We turn, then, to this focus.

ADOLESCENTS AS PARENTS

As noted in Chapter 2, the 1993 *Kids Count Data Book* indicates that when new American families are started by the birth of a new baby to a teenage mother, there is a major risk of experiencing problems such as living below the poverty line or poor school performance by the offspring. In other words, when the head of a family is an adolescent, the family and the children living in it have an elevated probability of experiencing financial and developmental risks. Unfortunately, there continue to be many American families headed by adolescents. Illustrations of the magnitude of this problem among contemporary adolescents include:

- Each year, one million adolescents become pregnant (di Mauro, 1995); about half have babies;
- Of adolescents who give birth, 46% go on welfare within four years; of *unmarried* adolescents who give birth, 73% go on welfare within four years (Lerner, 1995);
- By age 18 years, 25% of American females have been pregnant at least once (Lerner, 1995);
- Youth between 15 and 19 years account for 25% of the sexually transmitted disease (STD) cases each year. Moreover, 6.4% of adolescent runaways, of which there are between 750,000 and 1,000,000 *each year* in America, have positive serum tests for the AIDS virus (Lerner, 1995). These runaway youth often engage in unsafe sex, prostitution, and intravenous drug use. Thus, each year in America up to 64,000 "time bombs" are going out onto the streets of our towns and cities and spreading a disease that will kill them and the other people with whom they engage in unsafe sexual and drug use-related behaviors;
- About $25 billion in federal money is spent annually to provide social, health, and welfare services to families begun by teenagers (di Mauro, 1995);
- About 20% of adolescent girls in grades 8 through 11 are subjected to sexual harassment, and 75% of girls under the age of 14 who have had sexual relations are victims of rape (di Mauro, 1995). Thus, sex is usually forced among young adolescent girls (Carnegie Corporation of New York, 1995);
- Over the last three decades, the age of first intercourse has declined. Higher proportions of adolescent girls and boys reported being sexually experienced at each age between the ages of 15 and 20 in 1988 than in the early 1970s. In 1988, 27% of girls and 33% of boys had intercourse by their fifteenth birthday (Carnegie Corporation of New York, 1995);
- Pregnancy rates for girls younger than 15 years of age rose 4.1% between 1980-1988, a rate higher than for any other teenage age group (Carnegie Corporation of New York, 1995);
- In 1993 the proportion of all births to teenagers that were to unmarried teenagers was 71.8%. As shown in Figure 5.1, this rate represents an increase of 399% since 1963;
- Women who become mothers as teenagers are more likely to find themselves living in poverty later in their lives than women who delay childbearing. Although 28% of women who gave birth as teenagers were poor in their twenties and thirties, only 7% of women who gave birth after adolescence were living in poverty in their 20s and 30s (Carnegie Corporation of New York, 1995);
- In 1992, the federal government spent nearly $34 billion on Aid to Families with Dependent Children, Medicaid, and food stamps for families begun by adolescents (Carnegie Corporation of New York, 1995);

Family Diversity and Family Policy

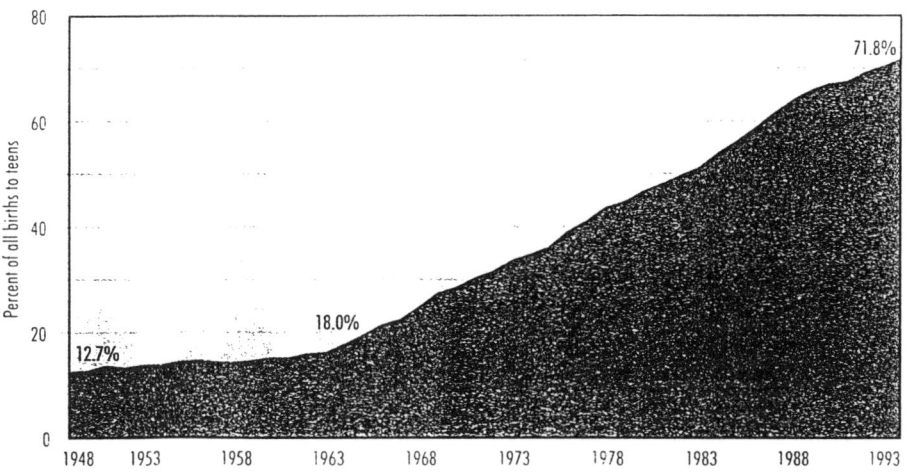

Figure 5.1 *Proportion of births to teens that were to unmarried teens, 1948-1993 (Children's Defense Fund, 1996; U.S. Department of Health and Human Services)*

- By the end of adolescence about 80% of males and about 70% of females have become sexually active. As shown in Figure 5.2, these rates represent significant increases across the last 15 years (Alan Guttmacher Institute, 1994; Carnegie Corporation of New York, 1995);
- Among sexually active female adolescents, 27% of 15- to 17-year-olds, and 16% of 18- to 19-year-olds use no method of contraception. Among Latino, African American, and European American adolescents, the percentage of females not using contraception is 35%, 23%, and 19%, respectively (United States Department of Health and Human Services, 1996);
- Among sexually active male adolescents in 1991, 21% report using no contraception at their last intercourse. An additional 56% of males used a condom and 23% relied on their female partner to use contraception (United States Department of Health and Human Services, 1996);
- By age 20, 74% of males, and 57% of females, who became sexually active by age 14 have had six or more sexual partners (United States Department of Health and Human Services, 1996);
- In 1991, 38% of the pregnancies among 15- to 19-year-olds ended in abortion (United States Department of Health and Human Services, 1996);
- By age 19, 15% of African American males have fathered a child. The corresponding rates for Latinos and European Americans is 11% and 7%, respectively (Lerner, 1995).

- However, 39% of the fathers of children born to 15-year-olds, and 47% of the fathers of children born to 16-year-olds, are older than 20 years of age (United States Department of Health and Human Services, 1996).

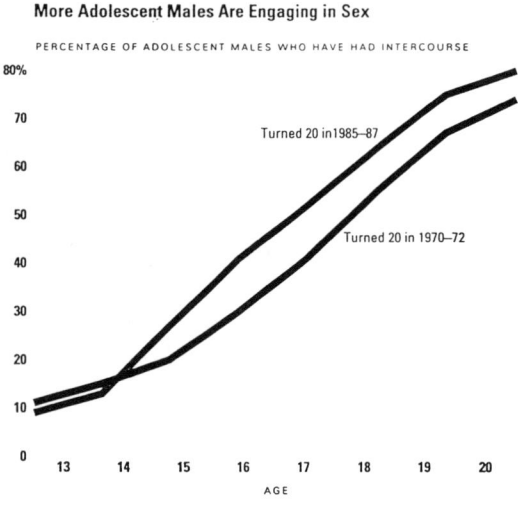

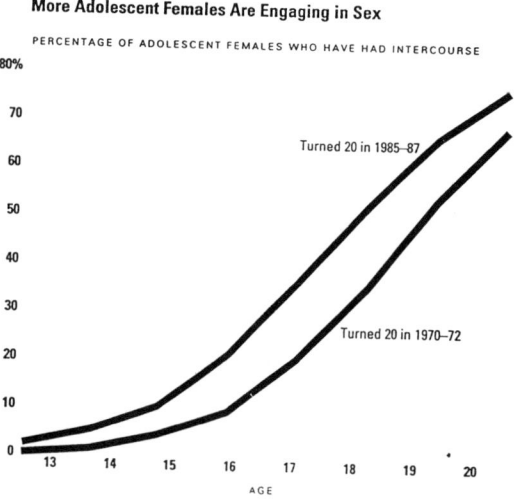

Figure 5.2 *Current cohorts of adolescents are more sexually active than cohorts of just 15 years ago: Percentage of adolescent males and adolescent females who have had intercourse by age and in relations to the dates in which they reached their twentieth birthdays (Carnegie Corporation of New York, 1995; Alan Guttmacher Institute, 1994).*

The breadth and variation of the above-noted problems pertinent to contemporary adolescent sexual behavior is staggering. The magnitude and diversity of the manifestation of these problems is challenging the educational, health care, and social service systems of America. The complexity of these problems is due at least in part to their connection to the other risk behaviors of adolescence and numerous individual and contextual influences on adolescents (Small & Luster, 1994).

To illustrate the several individual and contextual levels playing a role in adolescent sexual problems, we may note that biological, cognitive, and behavioral variables, and peer, family, and community ones influence adolescent sexual problems. For example, with regard to individual influences, ambivalent attitudes toward childbearing, contraception, contraceptive efficacy, and abortions are related to adolescent childbearing (Zabin, Astone, & Emerson, 1993). Similarly, possession of attitudes that reject societal norms, when combined with nonconforming behavior, is associated with early initiation of sexual intercourse among both African American and European American adolescents (Costa, Jessor, Donovan, & Fortenberry, 1995). In addition, among both male and female adolescents, poor psychological adjustment is linked to early initiation of sexual intercourse (Bingham & Crockett, 1996).

The peers of adolescents also influence their sexuality. For example, peer rejection in the sixth grade is associated with the number of sexual partners females will have over the next four years (Feldman, Rosenthal, Brown & Canning, 1995). In turn, however, peer acceptance, when it is associated with both a lot of dating and use of alcohol with classmates, is associated as well with the number of sexual partners adolescents have by tenth grade (Feldman, et al., 1995).

Moreover, the number of sexually active girlfriends that an adolescent female has, as well as the number of her sexually active sisters, and whether she has an adolescent childbearing sister, are linked to her possessing permissive sexual attitudes, having positive intentions for future sex, and being more likely to be a non-virgin (East, Felice, & Morgan, 1993). Thus, both peer and family contexts can combine to influence adolescent sexuality. This point is underscored by other research. Among African American and European American males and females, possession of a girlfriend or a boyfriend, respectively, one's educational expectations, and the educational background of one's mother were associated with being sexually active (Scott-Jones & White, 1990). Although these associations did not differ across the groups of African Americans and European Americans, it was the case that the former group of youth were less likely to use contraception than the latter group.

Family and peer contexts also influence the likelihood that adolescent girls will experience an incident of unwanted sexual activity (Small & Kerns, 1993). About 20% of girls report that unwanted sexual experiences have occurred within the past year. Approximately one-third of these encounters involved forced sexual intercourse; the other two-thirds of the events involved unwanted touching. Most of these experiences were initiated by boyfriends, dates, friends, or acquaintances (in this order). A girl's history of sexual abuse, a tendency to conform to peers, and having parents whose rearing style was either authoritarian or reflective of low monitoring were predictive of her being a target of an unwanted sexual advance. Similarly, in divorced families, a mother's dating behavior and her possession of sexually permissive attitudes influences both daughters' and sons' sexual activity (Whitbeck, et al., 1994).

The community context also influences adolescent sexuality. In poor communities, youth have higher rates of abortion and lower rates of marriage (Sullivan, 1993). In turn, among both African American and European American female adolescents, living in a socially disorganized, low income community where family planning services are not readily available is associated with the initiation of sexual intercourse and the young women's subsequent sexual activity.

CONCLUSIONS ABOUT THE PARENTING OF ADOLESCENTS AND ADOLESCENTS AS PARENTS

Parents are charged with an awesome responsibility by society. Through the family they create parents must develop the human resources—the people—who will carry society forward into the future. The children that the parents rear constitute this future. Society expects parents to do a good job, and create healthy and productive citizens. In most cases, parents fulfill these expectation. However, there are failures as well.

We have seen that parents vary in their rearing styles, the directions in which they socialize their youth, and the types of relationships they have with, and behaviors and emotions they show to, their offspring. A good deal of this diversity is not only quite healthy but is, in fact, necessary to maintain the richness of culture and experience that enhances human life. On the other hand, this variation—which can involve indulgent, neglectful, or authoritarian rearing styles, hostile interactions marked by negative emotions, and the display of problem behaviors—can result in significant problems for youth.

This diversity that exists in family functioning, coupled with the diversity we have seen to exist in regard to family structure, have pervasive implications for adolescent development. Families, in their structure and function, influence virtually all facets of the youth's psychological and social functioning. This influence may be associated with both positive and negative characteristics of adolescent behavior and development. As we have noted, all-too-often in today's society there are problematic outcomes of adolescents' relations with their families. In many cases these outcomes are associated with the adolescent himself or herself being a parent. Although family influences are not the only source of problems in adolescence, they covary with these other sources in affecting the incidence of problem behavior. At the same time, family of origin influences can protect youth from the occurrence of problem behaviors.

Indeed, insofar as the limits of scientific generalization permits, most youth have the personal, emotional, and social context resources necessary to meet successfully the biological, psychological, and social challenges of this period of life—either by themselves or as a consequence of intervention programs that may capitalize on their "plasticity" (Lerner, 1984), that is, on their potential for systematic development change (cf. Dryfoos, 1990; Hamburg, 1992; Lerner, 1995). Examples of some of the community-based programs that are indicative of this potential for successful interventions have been noted above. Such programs provide evidence that with a supportive social context attuned to the developmental changes and individuality of youth, healthy and successful people may emerge from the period of adolescence.

We have emphasized, however, that the challenges we must address to produce such positive outcomes on a more regular and sustained basis are more daunting when the developmental period of adolescence is coupled with the role of parent. As such, a key task for future scholarship is to identify the bases of successful development under such circumstances and, then, to translate such successes into appropriately scaled and sustained programs and policies.

Adults must adopt the ethos—once prevalent in communities but now more difficult to find—that *all* children in the community are *their* children. We must take the responsibility for preventing, and give each other the right to prevent, youth risk behaviors whenever and wherever we see them. If we "turn our backs" on our youth, if we do not work to extend the meaning and intent of effective, school-based programs to the entire community, and build a seamless social support net for our children and adolescents, then not only "their children," but "our children," and indeed all of us, will suffer in numerous and historically unprecedented ways.

The importance, then, of Schorr's (1988) idea that effective programs see children as part of families, and both as part of the community seems clear. Similarly, the truth of the now often-cited African proverb—that it takes an entire village to raise a child—has never appeared more certain. It will take the efforts of every citizen in a community to adequately protect their children and youth and, in turn, to increase to the level of absolute certainty the chance of every member of their younger generations to maximize his or her potential for healthy and productive development. We believe that through such an orientation we may best enhance the life chances of young people, especially when the life stage of adolescence coincides with the daunting duties associated with the role of parent.

6 THE IMPORTANCE OF DIVERSITY IN WELFARE REFORM

In 1996, Congress passed and President Clinton signed the Personal Responsibility and Work Opportunity Reconciliation Act (PRWORA; P.L. 104-193). This act replaced the Aid to Families with Dependent Children (AFDC) entitlement program, dissolved Emergency Assistance (EA), eliminated the Job Opportunities and Basic Skills Training (JOBS) Program, and substituted a single capped block grant for states, the Temporary Assistance to Needy Families (TANF) program, the funding of which is based on prior state welfare spending (Corbett, 1997; Zaslow, Tout, Smith, & Moore, 1998). The intent of this new welfare law is to turn custodial parents into breadwinners; public assistance is intended to become only a short-term phase of transition to self-sufficiency (Kondratas, 1997, p. 1).

Moreover, as explained by Morelli and Verhoef (in press, p. 4), the enactment of PRWORA:

> required individuals to work after two years of receiving federal subsidies; and set work participation requirements so that states must have at least half of the adults who receive . . . TANF working by the year 2002. Failure to meet this last obligation will result in states receiving less of the money allocated in their block grants. The legislation will increase the demand for child care among the nation's poor and near poor families, while at the same time decrease, in the long run, federal resources to provide these services.

That is, whereas PRWORA may enable welfare-to-work transitions among mothers, it may not enable them to provide quality child care to their children while they are making this transition. As a consequence, PRWORA may not afford healthy developmental transitions among children.

Families with children obviously have people in them at different points in their development and these people may, therefore, have a range of developmental needs. This range of needs may not be met by one single set of actions, or by a policy that did not take cognizance of the diverse developmental characteristics of the individuals—children, parents, or grandparents, for instance—that may exist within families. Thus, although, as Bogenschneider (1997) argues, "Welfare reformers face the dilemma of balancing two important, yet contradictory, goals—reducing family dependency on welfare, while enhancing or, at a minimum, doing no harm to the well-being of children" (p. 26), and the need to resolve this dilemma would seem to impose a two-generational approach on policy makers, the passage of PRWORA will make it more difficult to pursue such a multi-generational policy.

There does not need to be a zero-sum game mentality in thinking about how to develop multi-generational welfare policies. That is, despite the seeming contradiction in emphases—parent, or the family as a unit, versus an individual child—initiatives directed to parents do not have to be incompatible with actions aimed at enhancing their children (Bogenschneider & Corbett, 1995; Smith, 1995; Smith, Blank, & Collins, 1992; Smith & Zaslow, 1995; Zaslow, et al., 1998). For example, Nightingale and Holcomb (1997) suggest that welfare-to-work programs can be improved if participation is increased, implementation is strengthened, and ties to the labor market are built. A two-generation approach can facilitate this since mothers may be more likely to participate if there children are being looked after in high-quality settings. In turn, Bogenschneider (1997) notes that "Child development scholars have proposed two-generational approaches that also focus on parents' caregiving capacity, specifically their ability to support their children's development into competent, caring adults" (p. 26). Whereas it might very well be the case that such programs would really "end welfare as we know it," there seems to be a consensus among scholars of human development, the family, and welfare policy that PRWORA does not represent a policy that will move the nation in this direction. It will not facilitate both increasing the opportunities for mothers to develop skills and have experiences that will enhance their capacities for self-sufficiency, while at the same time providing quality child care for their children (Bogenschneider & Corbett, 1995; Bogenschneider, Corbett, & Bell, 1997; Bogenschneider, Corbett, Bell, & Linney, 1997; Morelli & Verhoef, in press; Smith, Fairchild, & Groginsky, 1997; Zaslow, et al., 1998).

Accordingly, in this chapter we argue that there is a failure to appreciate adequately in public policy the different developmental needs of the different (diverse) generations (children, their parents, and often their grandparents; for example, see Burton, 1990) involved in the social changes elicited by welfare reform. The failure to treat generational diversity adequately is one of the key issues raised in policy analyses pertinent to welfare reform. For instance, Zaslow, et al. (1998) point out that "The current legislation's focus on a rapid transition to employment rather than education or training suggests that there will be fewer opportunities to coordinate education and training services to parents with early childhood educational services" (p. 7).

Thus, not only is this new legislation potentially insensitive to the diverse developmental needs of the different generations comprising the family but, in fact, considerably more emphasis in policies discussion has been focused on the adult members of the family. Indeed, as stressed by Zaslow, et al. (1998):

> Much of the concern about the possible implications of the legislation has focused on adult recipients, especially whether adults will be able to make a transition to stable employment. . . . Yet children comprise the majority of those receiving public assistance. In 1995, approximately two-thirds (9.3 of 13.6 million) of those receiving Aid to Families with Dependent

Children each month were children. . . . Further, provisions of the new legislation, particularly the work requirements, have clear implications for children's child care situations and experiences within the family. Thus, there is also growing concern about how children may be affected by the new policy. (Zaslow, et al., 1998, p. 1)

Insensitivity to the developmental needs of children and thus to the importance of enhancing the lives of all generations living in poor families is a key instance of a lack of appropriate attention in contemporary welfare legislation to family diversity. However, as we will also explain, there are other instances of diversity that need to be considered as well in such analyses.

THE NATURE OF WELFARE POLICY: PAST AND PRESENT PERSPECTIVES

Children represent the human capital upon which the future of our nation rests. In turn, families constitute the essential component of America's *social capital*—that is, the links between individuals and institutions and, as well, among societal institutions—that support the positive development of children. Our social capital enables the life chances of children to be realized (i.e., social capital facilitates the optimal development of our human capital). Both the human and social capital of America are being threatened to historically unprecedented degrees (Lerner, Castellino, et al., 1995).

As we have emphasized in Chapter 2, poverty is the major factor linked to "rotten outcomes" (Schorr, 1988) of development for children and adolescents. That this linkage exists despite the enormous social interventions represented by America's welfare system suggests at least two points. First, despite where one is situated along our nation's political spectrum, one must conclude that past and, especially, current welfare policies have not produced the results desired from them. Second, one must also conclude that welfare reform must be undertaken to save our children, and thereby enhance America's human capital and social fabric. This is especially important because, as Bogenschneider (1997) notes, welfare benefits have not been sufficient to lift families out of poverty, and that the longer children remain poor, the more severe the effects of poverty on their development. Moreover, Bogenschneider points out that there may be negative effects of welfare receipt on child development that exist over and above those associated with being poor. For example, Zill, Moore, Smith, Steif, and Coiro (1991) found that while 47% of non-welfare poor children scored in lowest third on tests of vocabulary, 60% of children from welfare families were in this low scoring group, and only 27% of non-poor children were in this group. Smith, et al. (1992) report similar findings in regard to class rank and grade retention.

Simply, then, the nature of the contemporary problems confronting our nation's youth and their families requires that welfare reforms be instituted, and that innovative programs be derived from such policy initiatives, that focus on the positive development of *all* generations within the family. Unfortunately neither the history of welfare legislation in this nation nor the current policy context, framed by PRWORA, reveal adequate sensitivity to developmental diversity within families.

THE HISTORICAL CONTEXT OF PRWORA

Corbett (1997) notes that debates about welfare have been characterized by confused or confusing exchanges because the question underlying welfare has continued to shift across the history of legislation pertinent to welfare. As an example of these historical shifts, Zaslow, et al. (1998) point out that prior to 1935, private charity, or local and state government provided assistance to poor families. However, because the Great Depression created economic stresses (e.g., a 25% national unemployment rate) federal involvement in such assistance was needed. The Social Security Act of 1935 included the first national welfare legislation and created the Aid to Dependent Children program (which became the Aid to Families with Dependent Children in 1962). As also described by Corbett (1995), Zaslow, et al. (1998) note that child well-being was emphasized through this policy in that there was "a prevailing view that it was extremely important for young children to be reared at home by their mothers" (p. 3).

Similarly, Corbett (1997) indicates that whereas child well-being was the major concern of the policy makers who formulated AFDC, in the 1960s, policy concern shifted to income deficits and poverty. In addition, beginning during this same time period and continuing through the 1980s, interest shifted to labor market participation and private earning, and the welfare-to-work concept was regarded as the essential direction of welfare policy. Moreover, by the late 1980s, family formation and family stability became a focal concern, and discussions occurred about child support, the involvement of absent parents in this support, fertility (especially among teenagers), and non-marital births. Finally, by the mid-1990s, discussion about child well-being arose again, but perhaps in a different form or with a different tone. For instance, discussions of reinvigorating the role of orphanages was a part of the policy discussion during this period (Corbett, 1997, p. 11).

It is within this 1990s context that PRWORA became law. Characterizing this mid-1990s historical context, Corbett (1995, p. 1) observed that:

> Over the past decade (at least) we have witnessed major changes in the conceptual and political consensus that supports public assistance policy in the United States. In consequence, the nature of the policy has changed dramatically. The evolving consensus includes
> - renewed emphasis on the obligation of recipients of public assistance to seek employment and behave in ways consistent with an independent lifestyle;

- reorientation of welfare operations from an entitlement orientation to an emphasis upon the transition of recipients from welfare dependence to self-support;
- recognition of the role of services and support for adults both within welfare and outside welfare in facilitating the exodus of adults from welfare by means of employment; and
- appreciation of the importance of local public assistance agencies in the operation of welfare employment programs and as sources of innovation.

It was this prevailing set of ideas about welfare that enabled PRWORA to be enacted by a Republican-led Congress and signed into law by a Democratic President without serious political consequences for either major party. Indeed, Zaslow, et al. (1998) note that:

> The most recent legislation clearly reflects a national concern that policies should not foster, and indeed should discourage, teenage and nonmarital childbearing. Thus, views on the purpose of public assistance have changed dramatically over time. The earliest national welfare legislation had, as its aim, helping to insure that indigent mothers could remain at home to care for their children. The most recent legislation, in sharp contrast, requires that recipients work. (Zaslow, et al., 1998, pp. 2-3)

THE CURRENT CONTEXT OF PRWORA

Given the orientation to families represented by PRWORA, it is reasonable to ask how this legislation is impacting the structure and function of poor families and the lives of the parents and children within them. Unfortunately, the policy changes represented by PRWORA are too recent to have allowed a sufficient body of literature to have been amassed to address these issues (Zaslow, et al., 1998). Thus, scholars have extrapolated from existing scholarship about welfare—for instance, studies of mothers making welfare-to-work transitions, impacts on children, or risk and resiliency among welfare families—in order both to frame contemporary policy discussions and to provide a guide for future research.

For example, Zaslow, et al. (1998) discuss the findings of previous studies assessing the impact of welfare-to work programs in this way. They note that prior research has established the importance of understanding the diversity of welfare families (Zaslow, et al., 1998). They indicate that both risk and protective factors vary in welfare families. Such variation is associated with differential adult outcomes.

Similarly, child development outcomes vary also in relation to family diversity. That is, welfare-to-work programs influence multiple aspects of the family, and impacts on children will result from the combined negative and positive influences the programs have on families (Zaslow, et al., 1998). These impacts may range fully across a continuum from positive to negative. Moreover, Zaslow, et al. emphasize that individual differences in children, as well as variations in the programs experienced by parents, will be associated with variation in child outcomes. They suggest that:

> children may well benefit from the new policy if mothers successfully make the transition to employment and increased economic resources, particularly if the employment circumstances are not excessively stressful and child care is stable and of good quality. Children may also benefit from greater paternal support, both economic and social, if paternity and child support policies succeed in bringing about greater and more positive father involvement. Also, if work requirement and family cap policies succeed in restricting family size, children already present should benefit. (Zaslow, et al., 1998, p. 24)

However, other, less salutary outcomes for children are possible. Zaslow, et al. (1998) point to these as well:

> On the other hand, previous research raises the possibility that children in families in which the mother is less likely to make the transition to employment, in families that are more likely to come up against time limits, and in families that are ineligible under the new legislation already appear to be at greater risk for poor developmental outcomes. These children could experience negative outcomes as a result of PRWORA provisions.
>
> Finally, some children may experience neither negative *nor* positive cumulative effects of PRWORA per se, in that various policy provisions may well have small and/or offsetting influences. We need to keep in mind, however, that these children who do not benefit from PRWORA will likely remain at risk for the negative outcomes associated with long-term poverty, including poor health status, low academic achievement, and poor socioemotional adjustment. (pp. 24-25)

Other discussions of the import of welfare policy for children and families have also involved extrapolations from past research. For instance, prior to the enactment of PRWORA, Lerner, Bogenscheider, et al. (1995) discussed the key policy issues that should be considered in planning and enacting welfare reform. They underscored the need for policies to be designed, implemented, and evaluated in manners sensitive to the diversity of individuals and families involved in the welfare system. As we have indicated, this need remains inadequately addressed by the policy and program changes associated with PRWORA. As such, it is useful to consider the details of the Lerner, et al. perspective—with regard to policy perspectives pertinent to diversity that existed both prior to and after the enactment of PRWORA. The points raised prior to the enactment of PRWORA about the need to be more sensitive to diversity in welfare policy remain valid now, in the immediate years after PRWORA has become law.

POLICY DISCUSSIONS IN THE IMMEDIATE PRE- AND POST-PRWORA PERIOD

Just three years prior to the enactment of PRWORA, Corbett (1993) observed that for more than 50 years welfare in America has been associated with what was the most visible program of public income support for poor children, the Aid to Families with Dependent Children (AFDC) program. Indeed, Bane and Ellwood (1994) noted that conversation and legislation about welfare and welfare reform usually focused on this program. Moreover, they noted that while the AFDC program accounted for only one percent of total federal spending (e.g., in 1992, the AFDC program provided cash assistance to about 4.7 million families per month, at a cost to the federal government of about $13 billion), "it receives a much greater share of public attention" (Bane & Ellwood, 1994, p. x). Thus, as Corbett (1993) explained, welfare reform was usually discussed in terms of modifications in the scope, generosity, design, or administration of the AFDC program.

Accordingly, Blum (1992) discussed ways in which the Family Support Act (FSA), a federal law enacted in 1988, could help AFDC recipients become self-sufficient (i.e., leave the rolls of welfare). The FSA was aimed at enhancing the child support enforcement system in the United States, helping welfare recipients move into the labor market, and providing recipients with the services necessary to make a successful transition from welfare to work. To accomplish these tasks the FSA created the federal Job Opportunities and Basic Skills Training Program (JOBS). JOBS required states to develop welfare-to-work programs for welfare-dependent families, and the considerable policy discussion about this program involved, in the main, consideration of the capacity of JOBS to improve the employment status of AFDC recipients (Blum, 1992).

Although the JOBS program might have offered work opportunities to some AFDC recipients who had been unable to obtain employment, its impact on actually reducing the poverty rate among AFDC families was questionable. When it was developed, the JOBS program was based on an assumption that welfare mothers needed to work if they were going to be able to exit the welfare roles and become self-supporting. This assumption was faulty, since the facts indicated that even as early as the 1960s at least 30% of AFDC recipients worked before entering the program; and that another 30% combined work and welfare (Bane & Ellwood, 1994; Blum, 1992; Corbett, 1993). Combining welfare with work continued during this 30-year period and in 1994, four out of ten welfare recipients reported significant hours of paid employment during the survey period (Bane & Ellwood, 1994).

These statistics on the number of women who combined work with welfare suggested that among the population of recipients there had always been a subgroup that worked and who attempted to supplement benefits with wages. Yet, even for those women who worked, most were unskilled and received minimum wage. Their combined resources were not sufficient to raise them out of poverty, since in most states a minimum-wage job did not provide sufficient revenue to raise a family of three above poverty level. Thus, a program such as JOBS had minimal real impact on the status of welfare recipients because it was developed without an appreciation of the diversity that exists within the population and with little attention to the economic context. In addition to these complications, it is also worth noting that the FSA had never been adequately funded, especially the JOBS program and associated child care. Consequently, the promise of the program remained largely unfulfilled.

Welfare reform prior to PRWORA was also difficult to implement in a way that enhanced the lives of both the recipients and their children because it functioned within a social context that created a division between the "deserving" and "nondeserving" poor. The history of the AFDC program sheds some light on this occurrence. Originally, the program was designed to provide economic resources for mothers who were without a male breadwinner because of death. These women were considered the "deserving poor" and the state provided funding to enable them to remain in traditional female roles of homemaker and nurturer of children (Corbett, 1993, 1995a, 1995b, 1997). By 1935, the emphasis in the welfare program shifted from a focus on aid to mothers to providing for the children. It now provided grants for families headed by women who did not have male support, regardless of their status as widows. The program became more broad-based and the number of non-European American women eligible for benefits increased. By the 1970s, women of color (including a large percentage of African Americans), and divorced and never-married women became the majority of the AFDC caseload. When political conservatives began to attack the program in the 1980s, these women became the focus of the controversy (Corbett, 1993, 1995a, 1995b, 1997). The worthy European American widow that had characterized the public image of the welfare recipient prior to the 1940s had by the 1980s shifted to the unworthy urban African American woman and the negative stereotypical image of welfare mothers placed them in the public mind as the "undeserving poor" (Axinn & Hirsh, 1993).

Thus, the welfare reform efforts that were promoted prior to PRWORA were based on assumptions regarding recipients' willingness to work that had been developed with little consideration for the diversity within the recipient population or the economic conditions surrounding the program. The socially-constructed perception of welfare mothers as being the "undeserving poor" placed reform within a context that further complicated the development of effective policies that could actually bring about substantial changes in the lives of poor women and their children.

Moreover, Blum (1992) noted that "participation in a welfare-to-work program might create new problems for children by adding strains to family life or by exposing children to poor substitute care arrangements" (p. 1). Thus, Blum (1992) saw the need for policies that design "welfare-to-work programs that pursue the dual goals of economic self-sufficiency for families and healthy development of children . . . [that is, that pay] attention to children's need for nurturing parental support, a stimulating home environment that affords opportunities to learn, access to preventive health care, and high quality child care" (p. 2).

Accordingly, Blum (1992) cautioned that:

> if children's basic needs are neglected in welfare-to-work programs, the investment in parents' self-sufficiency will be squandered. Neither society nor individual families will be better off if parents are helped to move from welfare to employment, but children fail to attain the competencies they need to become productive adults. (p. 2)

Similarly, Corbett (1995a) noted that the "fatal flaw" in welfare policy prior to PRWORA—and, in his view, the key reason that child poverty continued to persist in America—was that:

> welfare is fatally flawed as an antipoverty strategy. That flaw is observed in the very concept of a welfare program. Basically, welfare programs are public transfers with two distinguishing characteristics: (1) the benefits can be received in the absence of work and (2) the rate at which benefits are reduced in the face of earnings substantially exceeds the rate we would dare impose on other members of society.

Both Kamerman and Kahn (1978) and Jacobs (1994) make comparable points. They discussed the difference between family policies that assist parents as "breadwinners" versus policies that aid parents in their roles as caregivers to children. "Breadwinner" policies enhance the economic viability of the family, through income maintenance or support for child care while parents work. "Caregiver" policies enhance family life and the development of family members. As Jacobs (1994) notes, extant policies in our nation greatly favor "breadwinner" policies.

Given the issues raised by Blum (1992), Corbett (1993), Kamerman and Kahn (1978), and Jacobs (1994), Blum (1992) called for a two-generational approach to welfare reform. As such, she raises for us what we see as the first, and arguably the superordinate, theme in our discussion of welfare reform and its implications for child and family policy and programming. This theme is one of four interrelated ones discussed by Lerner, et al. (1995).

WELFARE REFORM AND CHILD- AND FAMILY-PROGRAMMING: FOUR THEMES

Lerner, Bogenschneider, et al. (1995) noted that there are four key sets of ideas, or themes, that together define the innovations needed in welfare reform. These themes pertained to the need for welfare policy adopting a multigenerational perspective; the need for policy to embrace diversity, that is, to differentiate among the types of individuals and families on welfare; the necessity that welfare policy be developed in the context of knowledge about the dynamics of poverty and of welfare participation; and the need for welfare policy to recognize the diversity of single parent families.

As noted, although Lerner et al. were writing prior to the enactment of PRWORA, there is still reason to argue that these issues about diversity pertain to the post-PRWORA enactment era (e.g., Morelli & Verhoef, in press; Smith, et al., 1997). Simply, the nature and dynamics of welfare involvement prior to PRWORA may inform us about these features of welfare as they may exist under PRWORA.

Each of the themes noted by Lerner, et al. has important implications for the nature and development of youth- and family-serving programs. As noted above, these implications may be seen to arise most centrally because of the first theme, that is, the need for policies to promote an integrative, multigenerational approach to interventions.

Theme 1:   Welfare policy must use a multigenerational perspective.

Hernandez (1993, 1994) notes that most statistical studies of the economic status of children and families, and as well most public policies pertinent to these groups, focus on parents or adults as the unit of analysis (see, too, Jacobs & Davies, 1994). Indeed, Phillips and Bridgman (1995) note that:

> discussions of welfare rarely focus on children other than as family members who may benefit indirectly from their parents' improved economic status. There is scant information available about how young children are affected by their parents' welfare receipt or by transitions in and out of welfare, poverty, and work. Indeed, the research that has been done on the consequences for children of changes in family income yields little consensus as to how disparate trends in families' economic well-being affect children's development. (p. 1)

An emphasis on parents may be misleading if, through such a focus, policies fit to the needs of children are to be developed. For example, in 1988, while 27% of all American children lived in relative poverty only 18% of parents were in this economic status (Hernandez, 1993, 1994). In turn, at the other end of the economic spectrum, while 22% of all children in 1988 lived in luxury, 30% of parents had this status during this time period (Hernandez, 1993, 1994).

Simply, then, "the distribution of children's economic status can be quite different from that of parents or other adults" (Hernandez, 1994, p. 16), and welfare policies aimed at improving family circumstances for *both* children and parents must not make the error of focusing solely on parents. If the intention is to enhance the immediate and long-term development of both generations within the nuclear family, then policies must differentiate between youth and their parents. This is the case because policies "designed to enhance the welfare of families, parents, or adults may have quite different effects for children" (Hernandez, 1994, p. 19).

Zaslow and Eldred (1998) provide data pertinent to this point, at least insofar as the programs associated with such policy may be concerned. Zaslow and Eldred report that, among 290 low income young mothers (aged 16 to 22 years), a program (termed "The New Chance Demonstration," a national research and demonstration project that, between 1989 and 1992, was conducted in 10 states) that was effective in enhancing mothers' parenting behaviors had no positive influence on child behaviors presumably associated with their parenting. The affective quality of mother-child interaction and the quality of the cognitive stimulation mothers provided to their children improved as a consequence of program participation. These findings are impressive, especially because the mothers in the same studies by Zaslow and Eldred (1998) were at high risk for problems in parenting behaviors.

However, not all mothers profited equally from the New Chance Demonstration program. Zaslow and Eldred report that, despite being under similar levels of economic stress, there was diversity among the mothers in other background characteristics and these factors were associated with differential success in improving their parenting behaviors. For instance, mothers with higher literacy, more education, and better mental health and social support, and who also had children who had participated in child care were more likely to show improvements in parenting behaviors (Zaslow & Eldred, 1998).

Finally, however, Zaslow and Eldred (1998) report that although the parenting behaviors of mothers participating in the program improved, there was no association between this change and the cognitive and social development of their children, when assessed at 42 months of age. Zaslow and Eldred see this finding as indicative of the determination of children's behavior by the entire developmental system, involving not just the mother and her parenting skill but, as well, influences related to socioeconomic circumstances and the social and institutional relationships of both mothers and children, separately and together, across the breadth of the ecology of human development.

Accordingly, both the findings and their interpretation by Zaslow and Eldred (1998) underscore the point that a multi-generational intervention is need to enhance the lives of poor and low-income families. Even though one may have a program that is effective in promoting positive changes in one generation (the parental one, in the case of Zaslow and Eldred, 1998) a positive effect on members of other generations within the family (e.g., children) is not guaranteed.

However, Bogenschneider (1994) noted that much of the policy debate regarding welfare reform has been primarily one-generational, that is, it has focused on diminishing dependency among current welfare recipients (cf. Jacobs & Davies, 1994). While not denying the importance of this focus, Bogenschneider noted that an equally important emphasis is the children of welfare recipients and their future life chances and prospects.

For instance, Smith, Blank, and Collins (1992) pointed out that, by adolescence, 36% of AFDC children had repeated a grade, and that 23% of AFDC adolescents had been suspended or expelled from school. Moreover, Smith and Zaslow (1995) reported that young women who experience long bouts of poverty as children are twice as likely to be welfare recipients as adults.

Accordingly, Smith, et al. (1992), Smith and Zaslow (1995), and Bogenschneider (1994) have suggested that welfare reform would benefit from a two-generational approach which includes:

- Self-sufficiency programs, aimed at improving parent's employability through education and job training; and
- Child development programs, including preventive health care, high quality child care or early education, and parenting education.

Such reform will be highly innovative. For instance, Smith and Zaslow (1995) noted that until recently, few, if any, early childhood intervention programs have provided services to help improve parents' employability or, therefore, the likelihood that families would escape poverty. At the same time, programs of the past two decades that were designed to reduce welfare "dependency have either excluded women with young children, or paid little attention to the needs of children when these women did enroll" (Smith & Zaslow, 1995, p. 2).

Smith and Zaslow (1995) indicated that several recent models exist for programs that combine self-sufficiency services for parents with services aimed at promoting the positive development of children. Importantly, although sharing this commitment to a two-generation intervention strategy, the models discussed by Smith and Zaslow (1995) reflect, as a whole, a commitment to diversity with regard to: (a) the specific services provided to families and children of a particular community; (b) the types of families involved in the intervention; (c) the structure of the services delivered; and (d) the length of the intervention.

Thus, a two-generational approach to welfare reform would help resolve the fatal flaw of welfare policy discussed by Corbett (1993): A policy that provides job training or employment for a single mother may enhance the economic resources of the family. This will clearly benefit children since family poverty and low levels of maternal education are two of the most powerful predictors of children's success in school and social adjustment (Smith & Zaslow, 1995). Yet, Corbett (1993) pointed out that if the child is placed in an inadequate child care setting for 10 to 12 hours a day, while his or her mother is at or traveling to and from work, the potential problems of child development that may be produced may outweigh any benefits of increased economic resources for the family.

A two-generational approach to welfare reform would avoid such problems. From the perspective of Smith, et al. (1992) the components of a two-generation intervention are:

- Initial assessment of child and family needs, including appraisal of family circumstances that affect children's well-being, parenting strengths and concerns, the health care of the child and the parent, and child care;
- High quality child care and early childhood education;
- Provision of programs that strengthen parenting;
- Preventive health services for both children and parents;
- Provision of services that promote self-sufficiency and that lead to employment and to earning a living wage; and
- Case management.

The final element in this vision of a two-generational approach to welfare reform is important to emphasize because it underscores the significance of

Family Diversity and Family Policy

programmatic emphasis on the unique constellation of issues, capacities, and circumstances pertinent to a specific family. Indeed, a key feature of effective prevention programs is the provision of comprehensive and integrated services that are attuned to the characteristics of diversity pertinent to the individuals—the children and adults—within a given family, and we have noted that Smith and Zaslow (1995) pointed to the dimensions of diversity associated with various models of two-generation interventions. Indeed, this appreciation of diversity highlights the point that a two-generation strategy is an instance of a multigenerational orientation to intervening with children and families.

For example, as noted by Allison and Lerner (1993), Burton (1990), and Lerner, Castellino, Terry, Villarruel, and McKinney (1995), contemporary American families have a diverse range of structures. Some of this diversity involves children and grandparents or children and other relatives (e.g., aunts). Moreover, due to divorce, remarriage, adoption, and foster parenting, many families involve children and non-blood-related adults in parent roles.

As was illustrated in Table 1.1, the diversity of the contemporary American family underscores the need for an approach to welfare policy and to child- and family-programming that is aligned with this variation. To illustrate, it is useful to discuss one key programmatic issue affecting families on welfare: the need for quality child care.

Welfare Reform and Child Care

Phillips and Bridgman (1995), in a discussion of the influence of child care on the nature of child development, provided information that underscores the need for a multigenerational approach to welfare reform. Given the stress in welfare regulation that parents either work or participate in an educational or training program, that most non-working poor families (i.e., 82%) are headed by a single parent, and that most working-poor families (65%) involve two earners or a single parent (Hofferth, 1995), Phillips and Bridgman (1995) argued that one must consider "how children are affected by the care they receive while their parents are working or taking part in job training programs" (p. 17). Phillips and Bridgman noted that available research indicates that at most child care centers in the United States the needs of youth, and especially infants and toddlers, are not being met in regard to issues of health and safety, to positive social relations, and to cognitive development; these problems exist disproportionately for the children of low-income families (Cost, Quality and Child Care Outcomes Study Team, 1995; Howes & Smith, 1994). Indeed, 74% of children from such families had child care arrangements that were not safe, sanitary, or responsive to the child's needs.

There are numerous data sets indicating that not only does variation in the quality of child care have clear influences on youth development, with significant positive relations found between quality of care and child outcomes, but that the deleterious influences of poor care may be more pronounced among children from low-income families (Phillips, 1995). For instance, in a sample of 356 single mothers with children under age 13, Meyers (1993) found that mothers on AFDC were significantly more likely to drop out of the education and training program when they were dissatisfied with child care arrangements. Key aspects of child care that led to such dissatisfaction were lack of flexibility in accommodating sick children, low child-to-staff ratios, and lack of trust for the safety of their children.

Mothers who felt assured of the safety of their children and trusted their child care providers were twice as likely to complete the job training program as those who did not finish. Phillips and Bridgman (1995, 1997) believe that successful completion of job training rests on a reliable and acceptable quality of child care that fits parents' schedules, underscoring the key role that child care plays in facilitating work among poor families.

Moreover, Phillips (1995) stressed that there are problems with obtaining care per se when children are in their infancy or early school years, are disabled, have special health problems, and have parents with atypical or changing work schedules. In addition, for poor people, whose work patterns are likely to be more irregular than is the case for nonpoor people, there are problems also with obtaining stable, continuous care (Phillips, 1995). As a consequence, the already formidable problems that low-income families have in finding adequate child care are often increased.

Clearly, then, welfare reform policies must be developed in light of the impact of inadequate child care on the children of both the working and the non-working poor. In devising such policies, there are several key issues that Bridgman and Phillips (1996) noted need to be addressed by policy makers *and* by researchers interested in providing information engaging the work of policy makers. For instance the policy engagement process could focus on addressing questions such as:

> what factors guide state choices in spending child care block grant funds (e.g., budgets, political priorities, conflicts between political parties, the relative strengths of lobbying groups, the history of child care funding in the state) . . . how [do] state policy makers make trade-offs between serving welfare families and serving non-welfare families when both groups have low income, are working, and need child care assistance; between serving more families with smaller amounts of assistance or fewer families with more assistance; and between funding more child care subsidies to families and improvements in the quality of child care for low-income families. (Bridgman & Phillips, 1996, p. 17)

Blank (1997) noted some similar issues that require attention in the policy engagement process. She indicated that in the context of the implementation by states of the Child Care and Development Block Grant and the Family Support Act there has been an increasing focus on the consequences of shifting one's funding focus away from low-income working families toward either families on welfare and/or families in the process of making a transition from welfare. For instance, in 1994, half of the states and the District of Columbia increased the support of child care for welfare families rather than for low-income working families. Often, this was accomplished by diverting funds from the support of child care among the working poor to the support of child care among welfare families (Blank, 1997). Indeed, Blank noted that in many states there is an absence of understanding of the importance of assisting working poor families to provide child care.

Moreover, a paradox in the federal funding of child care must also be addressed in the policy engagement process. Phillips (1995, p. 34) noted that:

> The reduction of poverty has provided the most-long-standing rationale for child care policies in the Unites States. Nevertheless, federal child care subsidies are channeled disproportionately to the nonpoor.

For example, Phillips indicated that in 1993 more than 2.5 billion dollars in federal child care support were directed to the nonpoor (through the Child and Dependent Care Tax Credit) whereas only about 1.7 billion dollars were directed to the poor for child care (through the four main federal programs that serve the child care needs of the lowest-income families in our nation, e.g., the child care for AFDC recipients and the Transitional Child Care programs). Moreover, there is only one program (the Child Care and Development Block Grant program) that provides funding for improving child care. However, even with regard to this program, most money (78%) is directed to helping low-income families pay for child care and only about 9% is used to improve the quality of care (Phillips, 1995). Furthermore, Phillips (1995) emphasized that federal funding levels may constrain the capacity of states to contribute to the child care costs of poor families, and that states may not have resources sufficient to supplement federal money. As a consequence, the capacity of poor families to place their children in adequate child care may be further diminished.

Thus, there is strong evidence linking variations in the quality of care to differences in child outcomes or, in other words, we know that better quality care enhances the development of youth (Phillips, 1995; Phillips & Bridgman, 1995). Nevertheless, current emphases in policy do not manifest adequate appreciation of the distinct developmental needs of the diverse generations involved in working poor, in non-working poor, and/or in welfare families. Simply, then, as illustrated by the issues surrounding child care, welfare reform must attend to differences not only between children and parents but, as well, to the other dimensions of diversity that characterize individuals and families (Davies & Jacobs, 1994). This point raises the second theme in our discussion.

Theme 2: Policy must differentiate among the types of individuals and families on welfare.

Corbett (1993) pointed to the diversity that exists among our nation's poor people and, perhaps surprisingly to some, among the people who are dependent upon welfare. He noted that welfare dependent individuals are quite heterogeneous in regard to both personal characteristics and contextual or ecological circumstances. For instance, Bogenschneider and Corbett (1995) noted that the population of the economically dependent, rather than being homogeneous, can be clustered into distinct groups. For example, point-in-time estimates in the mid-1990s suggested that about two-thirds of welfare recipients were or would become long-term users of welfare. However, among new entrants into the welfare system, 30% were likely to use the system for three years or less and an additional 40% were likely to use the system for from three to eight years (Bogenschneider & Corbett, 1995). In turn, although it was estimated that 70% of new users of welfare would exit the system within two years, most (70%) would return to use the system within five years (Bogenschneider & Corbett, 1995).

One key implication of this diversity is that a monolithic, or undifferentiated, approach to welfare reform will not suffice either in enhancing the life chances of poor children or in removing adults from the welfare rolls. As such, Corbett (1993) argued that a key issue that policymakers must confront is how to differentially combine and implement particular policy options, from among the array that exist, in order to provide a "goodness of fit" (Lerner, 1995; Lerner & Lerner, 1989) with the needs and attributes of particular segments of the diverse people comprising the welfare dependent population.

One major reason for the difficulty in reaching consensus around welfare reform issues is a lack of consensus over the causes of poverty. For example, one view is exemplified by the "hards" (Corbett, 1993), those who contend that poverty results from personal failings, specifically differences in individual values and attitudes such as willingness and motivation to work. The "hards" often fix on an image of a welfare recipient as an African American teen mother who has dropped out of high school, does not work, and lives on public assistance.

An alternative view is exemplified by the "softs" (Corbett, 1993), who place the causes of poverty in institutions and structural factors such as low-paying jobs, poor educational systems, and unsafe neighborhoods. In a nutshell, the "softs" believe that if society provided good jobs and better living conditions, all people would be willing to work, and poverty and its associated ills would disappear. The "softs" envision a welfare recipient as a young struggling woman who is willing to work but whose personal ambition is thwarted by paternalism and/or racism, lack of job opportunities, low pay, and low quality child care.

Corbett questioned whether we need to choose one view over the other and proposed that "both positions reveal part of the truth, because no one image of the poor captures the full reality of this diverse population" (Corbett, 1993, p. 9). Thus, he stated that the policy lesson we can learn from this is that:

> no single welfare strategy, by itself, works particularly well. . . . The lesson is not that nothing can be done; rather it is that no single strategy will do the whole job. . . . [W]e must design solutions that respond to the diverse needs of the diverse population of the poor. (Corbett, 1993, p. 9)

Moreover, Corbett (1993) provided a conceptual scheme within which to begin to desegregate (differentiate among) the population of welfare dependent people. Using the metaphor of an onion, Corbett described several subgroups of welfare recipients. In the "outer layer" (of the onion) are those welfare recipients described

Family Diversity and Family Policy 95

by the "softs," the working poor and those people on welfare for less than two years. In the middle "layers" are those people with limited options and very low earnings capacities and have been on welfare for periods of two to eight years.

Finally, Corbett described the "core" of the onion, which may embody the characteristics described by the "hards." Here there are systems-dependent people (i.e., individuals with very low earnings capacity who, as well, have additional barriers to self-sufficiency, for example, chemical dependence or depression). The people in this "core" are long-term and chronic users of welfare.

Table 6.1
Corbett's "onion" model: The subgroups of individuals involved in the welfare system and the program options pertinent to them

SUBGROUPS	PROGRAMS FOR ADULTS	PROGRAMS FOR CHILDREN
OUTER LAYER Working poor and those on welfare for less than two years	*Foundation* Refundable personal tax credits Expand tax credit with cash value of food stamps Other tax reforms *Earnings* Earned Income Tax Credit (EITC) (index and base on family size) Direct earnings supplement Indexed minimum wage *Transitional* Assured medical coverage	*Reforms* Refundable child tax credits Assured child support *Supplements* Refundable child care credit *Supports* Assured child care
MIDDLE LAYER Those with limited options and very low earnings capacity (on welfare 2-8 years)	Welfare-to-work training programs Wage-bill subsidies Social contract Service options	Education reform "Soft" Learnfare School-to-jobs transition Youth capital account
THE CORE The systems-dependent: Those with very low earnings capacity and additional barriers— chemical dependence, depression, etc. (long-term and chronic users of welfare)	Work requirements Intensive services Time-limited financial assitance Guaranteed job	"Hard" Learnfare Teen pregnancy prevention Intensive services

Source: Corbett, 1993

Corbett (1993) pointed out that appropriate programmatic actions for individuals who are short-term recipients of welfare (i.e., those in the outer layer) will not be adequate for individuals who are chronically welfare-dependent (i.e., people in the core). Accordingly, Corbett (1993) suggested different welfare reform initiatives, for both adults and children, who are "located" in different layers of the onion. These recommendations are summarized by Corbett (1993) in a table, which is reproduced here as Table 6.1.

It is important to note, however, that the layers used in Corbett's onion metaphor are, in part, distinguished in terms of the length of time individuals within a layer remain on welfare. Thus, Corbett's (1993) conceptual framework pertains to the topic of the dynamics of welfare participation and, as well, to the study of the dynamics of poverty. A consideration of both of these dynamics is the third theme of our discussion.

Theme 3: Welfare policy must be attuned to the dynamics of poverty and of welfare participation.

As we have noted earlier (Hernandez, 1993; Annie E. Casey Foundation, 1997), the number of poor children in America has increased since the 1970s (see Chapters 1 and 2). However, despite this increase over the last several decades in the number of poor children, over the same time period the number of children dependent on welfare support (e.g., through AFDC) steadily *decreased* through the mid-1990s (Davidson, 1994). Between 1972 and 1987 the number of poor children receiving AFDC benefits decreased from 7.9 million to less than 7.4 million, and across the 1973 to 1987 period the percentage of poor children who received AFDC benefits decreased from 83.6% to 59.8% (Davidson, 1994).

Consistent with the differentiated response that we are proposing, some individuals who availed themselves of AFDC benefits used this support for a relatively brief period of time, while others received it for extended periods of time. For example, earlier we noted that Bogenschneider and Corbett estimated that 30% of the individuals initiating their first "spell" (i.e., period of time) on assistance were likely to be relatively short-term users, 40% were likely to be intermediate users, and 30% were expected to be chronic/persistent users.

Many writers have focused on the short-term users of welfare. For example, Gottschalk, McLanahan, and Sandefur (1994) pointed out that for a majority of individuals and families neither poverty nor welfare are a "trap," that is, a situation in which they are mired for extended periods of time and from which there is no escape. Indeed, this situation seems to hold for both parents *and* their children, that is, neither poverty nor AFDC participation by a parent irrevocably "sentenced" children to similar situations when they become adults.

Similarly, Gottschalk, et al. (1994) noted that most AFDC spells were short. For African Americans, for instance, "33.7 percent of spells last only one year, and an additional 16.2 percent of spells end in the second year . . . [while for non-African Americans] the corresponding figures are 44.0 and 22.8 percent" (Gottschalk, et al., 1994, p. 94). In turn, however, Gottschalk, et al. (1994) also noted that after seven years, 25.4% of the AFDC spells for African Americans were still ongoing, while the corresponding figure for non-African Americans was 5.8%.

However, although most AFDC spells were of relatively short duration, those individuals who did have long spells constituted the majority of people on welfare at any point in time. For instance, as explained by Bane and Ellwood (1994, p. 51):

> Overall, only 22 percent of those beginning a first spell stay for ten years, but that group represents 57 percent of recipients on welfare at a point in time. Similarly, even though only 32 percent of never-married mothers who begin on welfare will stay for ten years, we calculate that 66 percent of never-married mothers on welfare at a point in time are in the midst of total welfare time of ten years or more. The never-married mothers who move off more slowly tend to accumulate and become a much larger fraction of the overall caseload.

With never-married mothers constituting so much of the caseload at any point in time and, as well, with about 40% of AFDC spells beginning when a wife becomes a female head-of-household (e.g., through divorce) and with about another 40% beginning when an unmarried woman has a child, it seems clear that in most cases welfare happened when single-parent families were formed (Bane & Ellwood, 1994, pp. 54-55). As such, both policy development and programming efforts should be aimed at *preventing* the formation of such families, that is, at taking actions to reduce the probability of formation of single-parent families or the dissolution of two-parent families (Bane & Ellwood, 1994). Ideas pertinent to both possible policy innovations and programming options will be discussed below.

Here, however, it is useful to note that the nature of spells for welfare dynamics have been found to be analogous to spells involved in poverty dynamics more generally. Gottschalk, et al. (1994) reported that 59.4% of all poverty spells were of only one year duration, an additional 16.6% lasted for two years, and only 7.1% extended for seven years or longer. However, as with welfare dynamics, there were race differences: African Americans had longer poverty spells than did non-African Americans. While 63.1% of non-African Americans had poverty spells of one year or less, only 48.4% of African Americans fell into this category. In turn, while only 4.3% of non-African Americans had poverty spells of seven or more years, the corresponding figure for African Americans was about 15%. Thus, although there are important race differences, Gottschalk, et al. (1994) concluded that "a majority of the poor remain poor for short periods of time, and that a majority of welfare recipients receive welfare for only a few years" (p. 107).

Yet, other writers noted that while half of all new entrants would exit within two years, half of these would subsequently return to the rolls (Corbett, 1993). Thus, as noted above, at any one point in time, 60% to 70% of welfare recipients were or would become long-term users of welfare.

Bane and Ellwood (1994) found that five characteristics—race, education, marital status, work experience, and disability—were highly related to welfare dynamics. All of these characteristics were associated with length of a first spell and, as well, with the likelihood of recidivism (i.e., of returning to the welfare rolls for another spell after a prior spell had ended). However, Bane and Ellwood (1994, p. 39) noted that recidivism was more likely to occur in the first two years after a spell and that, if women stayed off welfare for three years, they were relatively unlikely to return to welfare. Accordingly, a sensitive period for programming may exist. If a program can help a woman stay off welfare for three years, recidivism may be prevented (Bane & Ellwood, 1994).

Moreover, insofar as race/ethnic differences are linked either to length of a first welfare spell or to recidivism, Bane and Ellwood (1994) found that, when factors other than race were held constant (e.g., educational level and family size), race differences were relatively modest. For instance, Bane and Ellwood noted that African American and European American recipients did not show major differences in length of first spells or in length of repeated spells (although there was a slightly higher recidivism rate among African Americans). Similarly, age of the youngest child in families receiving AFDC did not seem to be an especially strong predictor, in and of itself, of spell duration or recidivism (Bane & Ellwood, 1994).

Thus, extrapolating from these findings to the present welfare context, one may argue that programming should be aimed at mothers of children who are of diverse age levels. Focus only on mothers of young children may miss an equally viable opportunity to effect changes among mothers with older children (Bane & Ellwood, 1994).

Of course, characteristics such as race/ethnicity, age of youngest child, educational level, family size, employment history, marital status, and mother's age covary in the actual ecology of human development. Accordingly, it is necessary—both for policy and effective programming—to target this covariation in policy planning and program design. For instance, Bane and Ellwood (1994, p. 59) noted that "women with good education and recent work experience are much more likely to leave welfare for work." Accordingly, they suggested that programs that provide relevant educational experiences (e.g., pertinent to particular employment opportunities), coupled with programs that provide knowledge and skills pertinent to the work place, would seem to hold the promise of assisting women to leave welfare more rapidly (Bane & Ellwood, 1994). Although perhaps initially expensive, the potential of such actions to move likely long-term recipients of welfare to the work place would eventually result in both economic gain for the nation and human gain for the individuals and families involved in such programs.

Smith (1997), however, provided a note of caution. She noted that there are large numbers of American children who live in families wherein there is a substantial amount of work being undertaken by their caregivers that, nevertheless, does not result in freedom from poverty or near-poverty conditions. To illustrate, she noted that 18% of all children are in families wherein there is a full-year, full-time worker but, as well, a family income that is 200% of the poverty level (Smith, 1997).

Moreover, Smith (1997) noted that children in families that rely on welfare support and children in low-income working families are similarly at greater risk for problems of development and health than are children in higher-income families. However, children living in low-income working families do seem to have fewer

Family Diversity and Family Policy 99

behavioral problems than is the case with children living in welfare-reliant families (Smith, 1997).

Gottschalk, et al. (1994) also reported characteristics associated with spell duration and, as well, with the intergenerational transmission of participation in the welfare system. They noted that:

> It is true that individuals who lived in poor families as children are more likely to experience poverty as adults, and it is true that individuals who families participated in welfare programs when they were children are more likely to receive welfare as adults. (Gottschalk, et al., 1994, pp. 107-108)

However, they also indicated that:

> It is also true that as many as two-thirds of the children from these families manage to escape poverty and dependence when they grow up. (Gottschalk, et al., 1994, p. 108)

In considering, then, such diversity among welfare recipients, Bane and Ellwood (1994) drew a conclusion that has critical significance for policy:

> welfare is not a drug that ensnares the vast majority of people who ever avail themselves of welfare support. For most, welfare is a short-term transitional program. But for a smaller number, spells can be quite long. And these long-termers represent a very large portion of the recipients at any one time. (p. 36)

The interesting conundrum is that both perspectives, focusing either on short- or long-term welfare recipients, are accurate for certain segments of the welfare population, segments that change in response to fluctuations in the economy, to modifications in welfare policy, and to changes in local circumstances (Corbett, 1993). Policy responses need to be differentiated to accommodate differences in the will and ability of welfare recipients to become self-sufficient.

Referring once again to Table 6.1, those in the outer layer of the onion are those who have the skills, motivation, and necessary support to acquire economic self-sufficiency in a short time and who need only short-term support. Appropriate policy responses include time-limited economic support and short-term help in the labor market. Those at the core of the onion include both those with low-earnings capacity and also those who may experience psychosocial problems that interfere with their social values and capacity to work. Many new and proposed welfare reforms may apply to the hard core. For example, policy strategies for those with a tendency toward dependence might involve not only time limitation for welfare benefits, but also intensive services and guaranteed jobs.

The diversity of the dynamics of welfare underscores the points developed earlier in this chapter that an at least two-generation approach to welfare reform is necessary (children are different than adults); that reform must address the different types (or layers) of individuals involved in welfare; and that spells of welfare participation vary across various several demographic, contextual, or ecological categories.

Together, then, these points highlight the need for a much more differentiated, diversity-sensitive approach to welfare reform. Such an approach is predicated on adopting program alternatives from the array that may be available in order to match the needs, values, and developmental characteristics of the particular group of children or adults to which the program(s) are aimed (Bane & Ellwood, 1994). Simply, the differentiated approach to welfare reform forwarded in this chapter stresses an alignment between program elements and the diverse individual and ecological characteristics of children and families.

Accordingly, we are in agreement with the four policy "lessons" Bane and Ellwood (1994) derived from their research. That is, Bane and Ellwood (1994, pp. 65-66) indicated that it is important to:

- Recognize how dynamic and diverse the AFDC population is. Avoid simplistic stereotypes and the solutions they imply. One size cannot possibly fit all welfare recipients.
- Target those who will have long spells otherwise because they are where most of the dollars go. The poorly educated, those with little work experience, the never-married, and the young all deserve special attention.
- Not wait to see who becomes a long-term recipient, which mostly wastes time. And we find limited evidence that waiting until children reach a given age dramatically increases the ease of their mother's moving off welfare.
- Work as hard at keeping people off as one does at getting them off.

Bane and Ellwood recognized that following these lessons would not completely eliminate long-term use of welfare. However, they suggested that ignoring these lessons would certainly eliminate any opportunity to effectively diminish such use.

Thus, Bane and Ellwood maintained that there are potential pitfalls of policies that ignore—in either their design or implementation phase—the above-noted lessons and, we would add, the individual and ecological characteristics that we have discussed. A key instance of such policy problems occurs in the area of policy pertinent to single-parent families. This topic is the fourth theme we will discuss.

Theme 4: Welfare policy must recognize the diversity of single-parent families.

As we have noted, prior to PRWORA the most visible welfare program was AFDC, which sought to provide support for poor children. However, AFDC was not tied *directly* to children. Rather, AFDC was available primarily to single mothers and seldom when the father was present and unemployed. Access to other federal assistance programs for poor children, such as Medicaid, is often tied to AFDC eligibility as well.

Family Diversity and Family Policy

Yet single mothers are not a monolithic group. When couples divorce, only one of five mothers turned to AFDC (Seltzer, 1994), while about half (48%) of adolescent never-married mothers received some help from AFDC during the first year after the birth of their child (Committee on Ways and Means, 1994, p. 453). In 1992, 53% of AFDC recipients were never married; 30% were divorced/separated; 2% were widowed, and the rest were eligible for a variety of reasons (Committee on Ways and Means, 1994, p. 453).

While the proportion of single parent families has tripled in this country in the last 30 years (Seltzer, 1994), this is the first time in history that children are more apt to live in a single parent family for reasons other than the death of a spouse. In 1990, of the children who lived with one parent, 39% had parents who were divorced, 31% had parents who were never married, 24% had parents who had separated, and 7% had one parent who had died (Ooms, 1992). This means that children living with a single parent today most likely have another parent living somewhere else; yet, many welfare policies were originally conceived at a time when children lived in single parent families due to the death of one parent (Seltzer, 1994).

Little more than a decade ago, the conventional wisdom was that single parenthood had no long-lasting disadvantages for children. Recent evidence suggests, however, that children from single parent families do less well, on average, than children who grow up with both of their parents. When compared with two-parent families, children who grow up in single parent families are:

- Twice as likely to drop out of high school (McLanahan & Booth, 1989; McLanahan & Sandefur, 1994; Zill, 1983; Zill, Morrison, & Coiro, 1993);
- Six times more likely to be poor (McLanahan & Booth, 1989);
- Half as likely to find and keep a steady job (McLanahan & Booth, 1989; McLanahan & Sandefur, 1994); and
- Twice as likely to have psychological problems (Moore, 1992).

In addition, daughters from single parent families are three times as likely to bear a child out-of-wedlock (McLanahan & Booth, 1989; McLanahan & Sandefur, 1994) and more likely to receive welfare benefits as young adults than are daughters from two-parent families (McLanahan & Booth, 1983).

The consequences for children appear similar whether they live with a divorced or never-married mother (McLanahan & Sandefur, 1994). For example, early maturing girls in divorced families were more apt to be sexually active (65%) than early maturing girls in remarried families (54%) or in nondivorced families (40%) (Hetherington, 1993). Psychological problems are also three times more likely in children in remarried families than in intact two-parent families (Moore, 1992). Similarly, for adolescents whose parents separate or divorce, only one in five are able to maintain a good relationship with one or both parents during adolescence, compared with almost three in five in nondivorced families (Zill, et al., 1993).

Furthermore, single parenthood appears to disadvantage children regardless of sex, social class, ethnicity, or race, and appears to be related to lower child well-being among Cubans, Mexican Americans, Native Americans, and Puerto Ricans, but not Asians (Benson & Roehlkepartain, 1993; McLanahan & Sandefur, 1994). Nor does the age of the child matter much (Hetherington, 1991, 1993; McLanahan & Booth, 1989; McLanahan & Sandefur, 1994; Wallerstein & Blakeslee, 1989). In her earlier studies with younger children, Hetherington (1993) reported that parents and children adjusted reasonably well by two years after the divorce. Yet, in her most recent study, as the children aged into adolescence, those children who were previously functioning well started to show problems again.

Up until recently, policymakers and advocates have spent most of their efforts on developing programs and policies that prevent negative economic consequences for children who live with one parent. For the first time, however, some policy proposals have begun to address the option of strengthening marriage and preventing divorce (Ooms, 1992) and nonmarital births. Each of these will be discussed briefly.

One important recent direction that has received broad-based, bipartisan support is the effort to increase the private economic support available to children from noncustodial parents, primarily fathers. For children born out of wedlock, paternity establishment is one avenue for increasing child support. Before the passage of the Family Support Act, only about one of three children born out of wedlock had paternity established, even though 60% of unmarried fathers are estimated to be present at the birth of their child (Seltzer, 1994). Establishing paternity is important because it can result in child support payments and often provides access to other economic resources such as the biological father's health insurance.

Efforts to increase private child support payments by noncustodial parents, typically fathers, seem justified if one considers the amount of child support that is currently being paid to single parent families. Of all single mothers, about half are eligible for child support; of these mothers legally due child support, about half receive child support, and a fourth get no child support at all. Overall, about 60% of children with a nonresident father receive any child support. Of those who receive child support payments, the average payment is about $3,000 annually (Seltzer, 1994). Studies suggest that most noncustodial fathers could afford to pay more, but even substantial increases in child support payments will not remove children in single parent families from poverty (Seltzer, 1994).

Yet improving child support awards and enforcement remains an important strategy, not only for its potential to improve the economic well-being of children, but also because of its benefits for the children's emotional development. For example, children whose fathers pay child support exhibit better behavior and school performance. For reasons not yet known, evidence has suggested that a dollar of child support has a larger benefit on school outcomes than a dollar received from other sources, such as earnings or AFDC (Seltzer, 1994).

Thus, strengthening child support awards and their enforcement has the potential to benefit both children's economic welfare and emotional well-being. In keeping with the diversity theme of this chapter, however, the results appeared stronger for divorced than for never-married families. In general, welfare reforms that include child support provisions will benefit children, as long as they do not increase contact between highly conflictual parents. Based on visitation disputes in divorcing families, the number of families experiencing conflict are estimated to range from highs of one in five families to lows of one in 25 (Seltzer, 1994).

Furthermore, efforts to improve child support collection are more apt to be successful if considered along with increased attention to access and custody issues. Even though child support and child access are considered separately in the law, in practice they go hand in hand, and problems in one area are often associated with problems in the other (Seltzer, 1994).

Turning briefly to policy options of strengthening marriage and preventing divorce, the National Commission on America's Urban Families (1993) has sought to promote forming and maintaining stable two-parent families. This emphasis has been made in order to underscore the advantages for children of developing in a family with two parents.

This focus on the two-parent family structure should be expanded to incorporate the diversity among families highlighted earlier in the chapter. This is particularly the case within ethnic-minority cultures where the definition of "family" often includes extended-family members. In developing policies to support children and families that truly speak to the needs of all types of families, this cultural diversity must not be ignored.

While some argue that the high rates of divorce and nonmarital childbearing are private choices that government policy alone cannot change (Furstenberg & Cherlin, 1991), others cite several examples of how public education campaigns have successfully altered public attitudes and private behaviors around issues such as women's rights, smoking, AIDS, and the environment. While many marriage education programs have not been well evaluated, one program resulted in fewer separations and divorces, and fewer instances of physical violence in participating couples than among control couples (Renick, Blumberg, & Markman, 1992).

For those couples who do divorce, parenting education could enhance the ability of parents to "immunize" their children from negative consequences (McLanahan & Sandefur, 1994; National Commission on America's Urban Families, 1993). Some states have mandated or given judges the prerogative to require that parents in divorce proceedings attend a parenting class to learn of the impact of divorce on children and of ways to minimize its consequences. Few of these programs have been evaluated rigorously, but they appear to hold promise for cushioning the impact of divorce on adults and children (Furstenberg & Cherlin, 1991).

Finally, turning to the area of preventing nonmarital births, never married mothers have generated public attention because they are the most likely to be poor, to receive welfare for long periods, and the least likely to work (Ooms, 1992). Much of the public attention has been predicated on beliefs about whether public assistance is an incentive for adolescent fertility.

Corbett (1993) reviewed the several approaches to welfare reform that had been attempted by various levels of government. As noted, many of these approaches are summarized in Table 6.1. However, among the approaches not discussed in this table is one that Corbett (1993, p. 5) describes as the "make 'em suffer" strategy. This approach:

> refers to a broad set of proposals to impose penalties on what are classified as inappropriate or counterproductive behaviors. Benefits are conditioned on such positive activities as school attendance, partaking in work-preparation activities, immunizing children in the care of the recipient, not having more children while on public assistance, paying the rent, or avoiding certain felonious activities such as illegal drug use or dealing. (Corbett, 1993, p. 5)

In turn, of course, penalties would be imposed if these positive behaviors are not evident or, instead, if "negative" behaviors occur. In the context of this strategy, one such negative behavior would be childbirth while receiving welfare assistance.

This perspective is one that seems to reflect a lingering negative stereotype of a subgroup of welfare mothers who are considered by society to be "undeserving." Throughout the history of welfare, there have been efforts to control the behavior and reproductive lives of women who were considered by society to be irresponsible or inadequate mothers. In the early years of the welfare program, this was done through a "moral fitness" test where institutional agents determined the appropriateness of a woman's housekeeping, childrearing practices, and relationships with men before she was deemed eligible for benefits. These agents conducted intermittent home visits to assess the cleanliness of the household, and made what was known as "midnight raids" to insure that there were no men living in the house. Thus, during the early 1900s, a woman's family life and childrearing practices were inextricably tied to state support, and many women (mostly African American and immigrant) were denied benefits as a result (Abramovitz, 1988). The "make 'em suffer" approach is a modern-day moral fitness test, and once again, the parenting behaviors and lifestyles of a subgroup of welfare mothers are being scrutinized by society in order to determine their suitability for welfare benefits. On the surface, this approach may appear to be in keeping with the differential approach to welfare reform advanced in this chapter. However, it is more reflective of a systemic response to stereotyping, and represents a return to a time when women could be stigmatized and punished for what society determines to be "unacceptable behavior."

In other instances, however, the meting out of punishment for childbirth while receiving welfare assistance can have seriously negative effects for the community. This may be especially likely to occur if policymakers do not consider the range of individual (e.g., developmental) and ecological factors that may be engaged by a given punitive policy strategy.

For example, Wilcox (1994) noted that while the United States does have a teenage pregnancy problem, it is also true that the context of this problem is often not adequately appreciated and, as a consequence, that the policy actions pursued are ill-conceived and/or lead to unintended and undesirable consequences. Wilcox (1994) indicated that while it was the case that rates of unintended adolescent pregnancy remain unacceptably high—indeed, rates of adolescent pregnancy in the United States are higher than in any other industrialized nation (Hayes, 1987), increased over the past two decades and, as noted earlier, one million adolescents become pregnant each year in the United States—the rate of pregnancy among teenagers who have had intercourse has actually declined (Alan Guttmacher Institute, 1994).

Moreover, Wilcox (1994) noted that, contrary to popular belief, rates of adolescent childbearing declined from the mid-1950s through 1987, when the rates began to increase (Ventura, Martin, & Taffel, 1994; Vinovskis, 1988). In fact, the 1992 rate of 61 live births per 1,000 adolescents was well below the corresponding rates that existed throughout the 1950s and 1960s (Wilcox, 1994).

However, Wilcox (1994) indicated that policymakers have become concerned with demographic trends in *nonmarital* adolescent childbearing. The birth rate for unmarried adolescents has doubled since 1970 (Moore & Snyder, 1994), reaching, in 1992, a rate of 44.6 live births per 1,000 unmarried adolescents (Ventura, et al., 1994). Wilcox (1994) noted that policymakers' interest in this trend in births to unmarried adolescents derives from the results of several analyses of the burden placed on the federal budget by adolescent childbearing, and particularly nonmarital childbearing. For example, a report by the Center for Population Options (1992) estimated that the 1990 single year costs attributable to adolescent childbearing for three federal programs—AFDC, Food Stamps, and Medicaid—were approximately $25 billion! Moreover, Garfinkel and McLanahan (1986, 1994) indicated that the birth of a child to an unmarried adolescent mother increases the likelihood that she and her child will utilize programs such as AFDC. Indeed, Bane and Ellwood (1994) found that, in 30% of the cases, the beginning of a spell on AFDC was associated with the birth of a first child to an unmarried woman.

Wilcox (1994) noted that "a desire to receive welfare benefits" is one popular explanation for the rise in the number of households headed by unmarried teenage mothers. The argument was forwarded that the existence of AFDC and other benefits increases incentives for (and decreases disincentives against) teenagers getting pregnant and having babies out of wedlock (Murray, 1984). Indeed, the wide-spread belief in the validity of this explanation resulted in both federal and state welfare policy proposals being forwarded and, in some cases, policy actions being enacted. The rationale for these policies is related to the punitive "make 'em suffer" approach discussed by Corbett (1993). That is, the belief is that by placing greater constraints on the presumed welfare incentives for adolescent parenting, there will be a reduction in adolescent childbearing, a reduction in the number of people (mothers and children) on the welfare rolls, and a significant savings of tax dollars (Wilcox, 1994).

However, both research and practical experience proves this reasoning incorrect. For example, while Wilcox (1994) accepts the fact that it was possible that an incentive for teenage parenting existed within the AFDC system, he pointed out that it is not necessarily the case that the incentive was sufficiently strong to influence the behavior of adolescents. Indeed, reviews of research on this issue indicate that welfare benefits do not suffice as an explanation for childbearing among unmarried teenagers (Duncan, Hill, & Hoffman, 1988; Moffitt, 1992). Moreover, Wilcox (1994) noted that several demographic trends put this research into context. He indicated that only 15% of births to adolescents are intended, and nearly half of these are to married adolescents. As a consequence, only about 8% of all births to teenagers are births wanted by unmarried adolescents. In 1988, this trend involved about 37,500 intended births to unmarried teenagers (Moore, 1994). However, and again counter to popular belief, it was adult women—not adolescents—who accounted for the preponderant majority of both unintended pregnancies and unwanted births (Wilcox, 1994). In addition, the percentage of out-of-wedlock births to adolescents *decreased* from a level of 50% in 1970 to 30% in 1990 (Alan Guttmacher Institute, 1994).

These features of women's childbearing behavior once again underscore the need for diversity in welfare reform. Such reforms should take into account differences in the length of time women receive welfare benefits, and also differences in developmental stage of the welfare recipient. Furthermore, the effect of welfare benefits on the prevalence of single mothers appears to also depend upon family income. For example, Garfinkel and McLanahan (1986) contend that the increase in government benefits between 1960 and 1975 accounted for 9% to 14% of the increase of all single mothers and could possibly account for as much as 30% of the increase in the lower half of the income distribution.

Given these demographic trends and research findings, Wilcox (1994) concluded that it is not wise to build welfare policy around the fertility behavior of adolescents. Indeed, as noted above, there are examples of problematic consequences that may occur when such policies are enacted (Harris, 1994).

Harris (1994) noted that in 1988 voters in the State of Michigan approved a referendum halting the use of Medicaid funds for abortion. That is, beginning on December 12, 1988, Michigan taxpayers stopped funding abortions for poor women. As anticipated, as a consequence of the passage of this referendum the number of abortions decreased by 10,000 between 1988 and 1989, dropping from 45,000 to 35,000 (Harris, 1994).

In turn, however, over this same period the number of births to teenagers increased by over 10%, from 17,000 to over 19,000; the number of low birth-weight babies increased by 10%; and the number of infants born with congenital anomalies increased by over 400%, from 746 to 3,161 (Harris, 1994).

Particular communities where there may be a higher proportion of poor people may be especially affected by such punitive policy strategies. Again, data from Michigan underscore this possibility. Before enactment of the 1988 referendum, 20% of all births in Detroit were to teenagers; after enactment this rate rose to 25% (Harris, 1994). In addition, Detroit experienced an increase of 54% in births to mothers who did not receive adequate prenatal care and, in turn, an increase of 33% in low birth-weight infants (Harris, 1994).

Accordingly, while the punitive policy approved by Michigan voters did result in a marked decrease in number of abortions, there have also been negative social and economic consequences. Arguably, failure to adopt a differentiated, diversity-sensitive approach to welfare reform can result in exacerbation of some of the problems that a strategy was intended to reduce. In the view of Lerner, Bogenschneider, et al. (1995), such differentiation is needed, particularly in that this conception of reform includes quite centrally the idea of differentiation in respect to a two-generational strategy, or better, a multigenerational strategy. Indeed, Bogenschneider and Corbett (1995) see the development of such a strategy as perhaps the key element of a diversity-sensitive reform of welfare policy. They state that:

> Welfare reform might benefit from a two generational approach—breadwinner strategies designed to improve parents' employability and self-sufficiency, and caregiving strategies which improve parents' abilities to promote [e.g., through high quality child care; Phillips, 1995] children's well-being. (Bogenschneider & Corbett, 1995, p. 41; bracketed material added by the present authors)

Bogenschneider and Corbett went on to note that the:

> next issue on the agenda may be three-generational models which focus on the needs of children, parents, and grandparents. . . . Also two-generational models may need to be defined broadly to include whoever cares for the child. For example, mothers on AFDC often have men in their lives who can be a powerful untapped force for family improvement. (Bogenschneider & Corbett, 1995, p. 42)

In fact, Bogenschneider, Ragsdale, and Linney (1995) believe that federal and state policy reforms that strengthen men's financial and interpersonal ties to their biological or adopted children, but that safeguard the child against the problems of increased embeddedness in highly conflictual parental interactions—for example, that may exist after a divorce—can enhance children's economic welfare and social and emotional well-being.

In short, then, Bogenschneider, Corbett, and their colleagues call for policy innovations that are attentive to the rich and complex interpersonal and generational diversity present among poor families. The importance of policies predicated on such developmental diversity is a theme associated with the third illustration of the role of developmental contextualism in policy development: youth policy that promotes positive development.

7 TOWARD THE DEVELOPMENT OF A NATIONAL YOUTH POLICY

Children constitute 100% of the future human and social capital upon which our nation must depend. The healthy rearing of children has often been identified as the essential function of the family (Bowman & Spanier, 1978; Lerner & Spanier, 1980). As such, although family policy is not isomorphic with child or youth policy (e.g., family policies may involve aged adults living in retirement and without children or grandchildren), it is arguably the case that there are no policy issues of greater concern to America's families than those that pertain to the health or welfare of their children.

In Chapter 1, we stressed the view that society has charged the family with the primary responsibility for rearing children, and maintained that the family was "invented" as the institution that could best raise children in a safe, healthy, and effective manner—that is, with effectiveness, operationalized—both historically and in an evolutionary sense (Johanson & Edey, 1981; Lerner, 1984; Lerner & Spanier, 1978, 1980)—as producing citizens committed to the maintenance and perpetuation of society. The family, then, is the key institution contributing to civil society (Lerner, 1984; Lerner & Spanier, 1978, 1980), and—in this sense—*family policies represent societal principles or strategies for furthering civil society through the nurturance and socialization of children by families.* If families are effective institutions, children will become productive and committed members of society.

Nevertheless, despite the crucial connection between families, children, and civil society, it is still the case that, today, all too many Americans do not see the need for a comprehensive and integrated national policy pertinent to all of our nation's children. To the contrary, many Americans see youth problems as associated with other people's children. Their stereotyped image of the "at-risk" or poor child is of a minority youth living in the inner city. Yet, the probability that an American child or adolescent will be poor—and thus experience the several "rotten outcomes" (Schorr, 1988) of poverty—does not differ with regard to whether that youth lives in an urban or rural setting (Huston, 1991). Moreover, the incidence of risk behaviors among our nation's youth (Dryfoos, 1990, 1994) extends the problems of America's children and adolescents far beyond the bounds associated with the numbers of our nation's poor or minority children.

For these reasons alone there appears to be ample reason for the development of a national youth policy pertinent to all of America's children and adolescents. However, there are additional reasons. Just as we may be concerned with developing better policies for sustaining and/or enhancing American agricultural, industrial, manufacturing, and business interests, it would seem clear that we must not lose sight of the need to sustain the communities—and the people—involved in the production, distribution, *and* consumption of the products of our economy.

Still, we often neglect the fact that problems of rural and urban youth—problems that are similarly structured, similarly debilitating, and similarly destructive of America's human capital—diminish significantly our nation's present and future ability to sustain and enhance our nation's economic productivity. Clearly, then, both from the standpoint of the problems of children and adolescents, and from the perspective of enlightened self-interest within America's industrial, agricultural, business, and consumer communities, policies need to be directed to enhancing youth development, and preventing the loss of human capital associated with the breadth and depth of the problems confronting our children and youth.

PROBLEMS RESULTING FROM THE ABSENCE OF A NATIONAL YOUTH POLICY

Despite the historically unprecedented growth in the magnitude of the problems of America's youth, and the contextual conditions that exacerbate these problems (e.g., changes in family structure and function, and in child and adolescent poverty rates—described in Chapters 1 and 2), there have been few major policy initiatives taken to address these increasingly more dire circumstances. Indeed, as Hamburg (1992, p. 13) has noted:

> During the past three decades, as all these remarkable changes increasingly jeopardized healthy child development, the nation took little notice. One arcane but important manifestation of this neglect was the low research priority and inadequate science policy for this field. As a result, the nature of this new generation of problems was poorly understood; emerging trends were insufficiently recognized; and authority tended to substitute for evidence, and ideology for analysis. Until the past few years, political, business, and professional leaders had very little to say about the problems of children and youth. Presidents have tended to pass the responsibility to the states and the private sector. State leaders often passed the responsibility back to the federal government on the one hand or over to the cities on the other. And so it goes.

As a result of this "treatment" of social policy regarding our nation's children and adolescents, the United States has no national youth policy per se (Hahn, 1994). Rather, policies, and the programs associated with them, tend to be focused only on the family [e.g., Aid for Dependent Children (AFDC) or the Personal Responsibility and Work Opportunity Reconciliation Act (PRWORA)] and not on youth per se (Corbett, 1995; Huston, 1991; Morelli & Verhoef, in press; Zaslow, et al., 1998).

Family Diversity and Family Policy

As such, while these policies may influence the financial status of the family, they may not readily impact on, and certainly they fail to emphasize, youth development. That is, these policies do not focus on the enhancement of the capacities and the potentials of America's children and adolescents. For instance, as we have suggested in Chapter 6, a policy or program that provides a job for an unemployed single mother, but results in the placement of her child in an inadequate day care environment for extended periods of time, may enhance the financial resources of the family but it may do so at the cost of placing the child in an unstimulating and, possibly, detrimental environment.

Accordingly, if we are to substantially reduce the current waste of human life and potential caused by the problems confronting contemporary American youth, new policy options must be pursued, ones that focus on children and adolescents and emphasize not only amelioration, remediation, and/or deterrence of problems, but positive youth development as well. Thus, as argued by Pittman and Zeldin (1994, p. 53):

> The reduction of problem behaviors among young people is a necessary policy goal. But it is not enough. We must be equally committed to articulating and nurturing those attributes that we wish adolescents to develop and demonstrate.

THE PROMOTION OF DEVELOPMENTAL ASSETS

What is required for the promotion of positive development in our nation's young people? Peter L. Benson and his colleagues at the Search Institute in Minneapolis believe that what is needed is the application of "assets" (Benson, 1997; Benson, Leffert, Scales, & Blyth, 1998; Leffert, Benson, Scales, Sharma, Drake, & Blyth, 1998; Scales & Leffert, 1999). They stress that positive youth development is furthered when actions are taken to enhance the strengths of a person (e.g., a commitment to learning, a healthy sense of identity), a family (e.g., caring attitudes toward children, rearing styles that both empower youth and set boundaries and provide expectations for positive growth), and a community (e.g., social support, programs that provide access to the resources for education, safety, and mentorship available in a community) (Benson, 1997).

Accordingly, Benson and his colleagues believe there are both internal and external attributes that comprise the developmental assets needed by youth. Through their research they have identified 40 such assets, 20 internal ones and 20 external ones. These attributes are presented in Table 7.1.

Benson and his colleagues have found that the more developmental assets possessed by an adolescent the greater the likelihood of his or her positive, healthy development. For instance, in a study of 99,462 youth in Grades 6 through 12 in public and/or alternative schools from 213 cities and town in the United States who were assessed during the 1996-97 academic year for their possession of the 40 assets

Table 7.1 *40 Developmental Assets*

External	*Support*	1.	*Family support*—Family life provides high levels of love and support.
		2.	*Positive family communication*—Young person and his or her parent(s) communicate positively, and young person is willing to seek advice and counsel from parent(s).
		3.	*Other adult relationships*—Young person receives support from three or more nonparent adults.
		4.	*Caring neighborhood*—Young person experiences caring neighbors.
		5.	*Caring school climate*—School provides a caring, encouraging environment
		6.	*Parent involvement in schooling*—Parent(s) are actively involved in helping young person succeed in school.
	Empowerment	7.	*Community values youth*—Young person perceives that adults in the community value youth.
		8.	*Youth as resources*—Young people are given useful roles in the community.
		9.	*Service to others*—Young person serves in the community one hour or more per week.
		10.	*Safety*—Young person feels safe in home, at school, and the neighborhood.
	Boundaries and Expectations	11.	*Family boundaries*—Family has clear rules and consequences and monitors the young person's whereabouts.
		12.	*School boundaries*—School provides clear rules and consequences.
		13.	*Neighborhood boundaries*—Neighbors take responsibility for monitoring young people's behavior.
		14.	*Adult role models*—Parent(s) and other adult model positive, responsible behavior.
		15.	*Positive peer influence*—Young person's best friends model positive, responsible behavior.
		16.	*High expectations*—Both parent(s) and teachers encourage the young person to do well.
	Constructive Use of Time	17.	*Creative activities*—Young person spends three or more hours per week in lessons or practice in music, theater, or other arts.
		18.	*Youth programs*—Young person spends three hours or more per week in sports, clubs, or organizations at school and/or in community organizations.
		19.	*Religious community*—Young person spends one or more hours per week in activities in a religious institution.
		20.	*Time at home*—Young person is out with friends "with nothing special to do" two or fewer nights per week.

Internal	Commitment to Learning	21. *Achievement motivation*—Young person is motivated to do well in school. 22. *School engagement*—Young person is actively engaged in learning. 23. *Homework*—Young person reports doing at least one hour of homework every school day. 24. *Bonding to school*—Young person cares about his or her school. 25. *Reading for pleasure*—Young person reads for pleasure three or more hours per week.
	Positive Values	26. *Caring*—Young person places high value on helping other people. 27. *Equality and social justice*—Young person places high value on promoting equality and reducing hunger and poverty. 28. *Integrity*—Young person acts on convictions and stands up for her or his beliefs. 29. *Honesty*—Young person "tells the truth even when it is not easy." 30. *Responsibility*—Young person accepts and takes personal responsibility. 31. *Restraint*—Young person believes it is important not to be sexually active or to use alcohol or other drugs.
	Social Competencies	32. *Planning and decision making*—Young person knows how to plan ahead and make choices. 33. *Interpersonal competence*—Young person has empathy, sensitivity, and friendship skills. 34. *Cultural competence*—Young person has knowledge of and comfort with people of different cultural/racial/ethnic backgrounds. 35. *Resistance skills*—Young person can resist negative peer pressue and dangerous situations. 36. *Peaceful conflict resolution*—Young person seeks to resolve conflict nonviolently.
	Positive Identity	37. *Personal power*—Young person feels he or she has control over "things that happen to me." 38. *Self-esteem*—Young person reports having high self-esteem. 39. *Sense of purpose*—Young person reports that "my life has a purpose." 40. *Positive view of personal future*—Young person is optimistic about her or his personal future.

Source: Benson, et al., 1998

presented in Table 7.1, Leffert, et al. (1998) found that the more assets present among youth the lower the likelihood of alcohol use, depression/suicide risk, and violence. Figures 7.1, 7.2, and 7.3, taken from the research of Leffert, et al., present these findings.

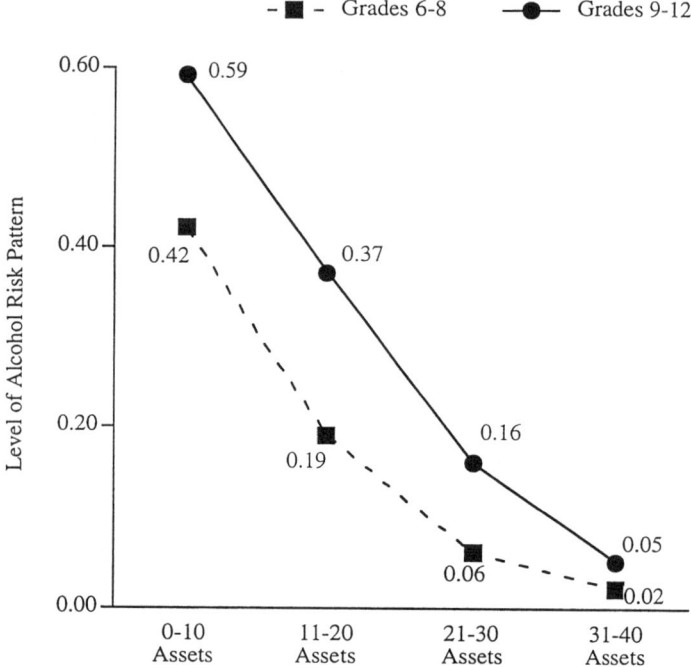

Figure 7.1 *The effect of Grade x Asset Level interaction on alcohol risk pattern (Leffert, et al., 1998)*

For instance, Figure 7.1 displays the level of alcohol use risk for youth in Grades 6-8 combined and for youth in Grades 9-12 combined. As shown in this figure in both grade groupings alcohol risk decreases with the possession of more assets. Youth with zero to 10 assets have the highest risk, followed by youth with 11 to 20 assets, youth with 21 to 30 assets, and youth with 31 to 40 assets. Thus, consistent with Benson's (1997) view of the salience of developmental assets for promoting healthy behavior among young people, both the trend lines represented in the figure, and the fact that the last group has the lowest level of risk, shows the importance of the asset approach in work aimed at promoting positive development in our nation's children and adolescents. Moreover, the data summarized in both Figures 7.2 and 7.3 replicate the trends seen in Figure 7.1—for males and females in regard to depression/suicide risk in the case of Figure 7.2 and for combinations of males and females in different grade groupings in regard to violence risk in the case of Figure 7.3. This congruence strengthens the argument for the critical significance of a focus on developmental assets in public policy discussions about building a national youth policy aimed at the promotion of positive youth development.

There are other data sets that support the importance of focusing on developmental assets in both understanding the bases of positive youth development and using that knowledge to inform the policy-making process. Luster and McAdoo (1994) sought to identify the factors that contribute to individual differences in the

Family Diversity and Family Policy

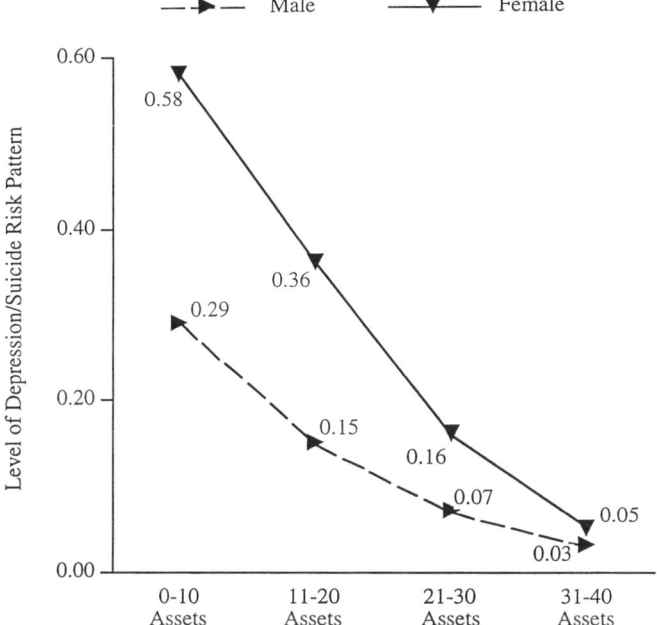

Figure 7.2 *The effect of Sex x Asset Level interaction on depression and suicide risk pattern (Leffert, et al., 1998)*

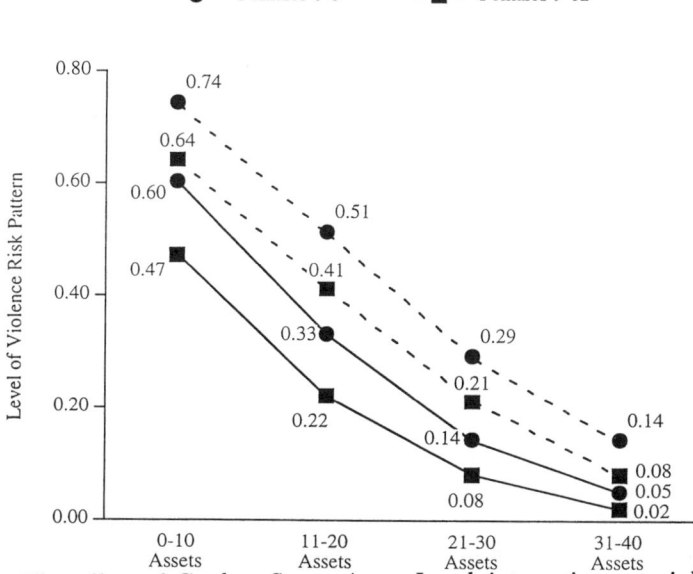

Figure 7.3 *The effect of Grade x Sex x Asset Level interaction on violence risk pattern (Leffert, et al., 1998)*

cognitive competence of African American children in the early elementary grades. Using data from the National Longitudinal Study of Youth (NLSY), and consistent with an asset-based approach to promoting the positive development of youth (Benson, 1997; Scales & Leffert, 1999), they found that favorable outcomes in cognitive and socioemotional development (operationalized as attainments within the top quartile of the sample they studied) were associated with high scores on an "advantage index." This index was formed by scoring children on the basis of the absence of risk factors (e.g., pertaining to poverty or problems in the quality of the home environment) and the presence of more favorable circumstances in their lives.

As an illustration of their findings, Luster and McAdoo (1994) report that, whereas only 4% of the children in their sample who scored low on the advantage index had high scores on a measure of vocabulary, 44% of the children who had high scores on the measure of developing under favorable circumstances also had high vocabulary scores. Similar contrasts between low and high scorers on the advantage index were found in measures of math achievement (14% versus 37%, respectively), word recognition (0% versus 35%, respectively), and word meaning (7% and 46%, respectively).

Findings reported by Luster and McAdoo (1996) extend those of Luster and McAdoo (1994). Seeking to identify the factors that contribute to individual differences in the educational attainment of African American young adults from low socioeconomic status, Luster and McAdoo (1996) found that assets associated with the individual (cognitive competence, academic motivation, and personal adjustment in kindergarten) and the context (parental involvement in schools) were associated longitudinally with academic achievement and educational attainment.

In short, the individual and contextual assets of youth are linked to their positive development. These data legitimate the idea that the enhancement of such assets will be associated with the promotion of positive youth development. Consistent with the perspective forwarded by Benson (1997), and the data provided by Leffert, et al. (1998) and by Luster and McAdoo (1994, 1996), Pittman and Zeldin (1994) forward several policy recommendations that provide a frame for us to discuss the development of a national youth policy supportive of the positive development of children and adolescents.

POTENTIAL DIMENSIONS OF A NATIONAL YOUTH POLICY

Both Benson (1997) and Pittman and Zeldin (1994) emphasize that policy must focus on promoting positive features of youth development, and not on the deterrence of negative characteristics. As described by Benson (1997), assets must be marshaled to promote the competencies and potentials of youth, and develop and evaluate programs designed to promote these positive attributes. Accordingly, policy must go beyond two necessary but not sufficient goals—first, of "meeting basic human needs [through ensuring] economic security, food, shelter, good and useful work, and safety" (Benson, 1997, p. xiii) for youth and the members of their families; and second, targeting and reducing, or even eliminating "the risks and deficits that diminish or thwart the healthy development of children and adolescents.

Family Diversity and Family Policy 117

Guns, unsafe streets, predatory adults, abuse, family violence, exclusion, alcohol and other drugs, racism, and sexism are among the threats" (Benson, 1997, pp. xiii-xiv). Policy must add the third component—of assets—that is crucial for building a strong young person supported through positive relationships with his/her family and community. Indeed, as Benson, et al. (1998, p. 156) note:

> Ultimately, the most critical question is how communities can be supported to integrate and simultaneously pursue strength-building in three community infrastructures: economic, service delivery, and development. The goal of this integration is to develop a combination of policy, resources, and actions which will meet basic human needs, reduce threats to human development, provide humane and effective access to services, and promote healthy development.

The work of Benson and his colleagues provides a vision for a new direction in American public policy, one that has been brought to the fore by such recent events as the April 1997 Presidents' Summit in Philadelphia. Here, all living American Presidents forwarded a vision for the development of policy that would provide every youth in America with nurturance from at least one adult committed unconditionally to the welfare and positive development of the child; a healthy life start for all young people; a safe environment within which to live; the opportunity to have an education that will result in the attainment of marketable skills; and the inculcation of values for and opportunities to "give back" to others, that is, to volunteer to serve the community.

A MODEL OF A NATIONAL YOUTH POLICY

Together, then, the ideas of developmental assets and of promoting positive youth development coalesce to provide a framework for a model of a national youth policy. Supplemented by ideas pertinent to what constitutes the outcomes for individuals of positive youth development (Carnegie Council on Adolescent Development, 1989; Lerner, 1995; Little, 1993), this model rests on the ideas we have presented about the function of the family in society, that is, that civil society is furthered through the family's effective nurturance and socialization of children. This model of youth policy that derives from this tripartite emphasis on families, children, and civil society is presented in Figure 7.4.

As shown in the figure, public policies should be aimed at insuring that families have the capacity to provide for children: boundaries and expectations; fulfillment of physiological and safety needs; a climate of love and caring; the inculcation of self-esteem; the encouragement for growth; positive values; and positive links to the community. The programs that derive from these policies should insure that the resources that families need to nurture and socialize children in these manner are available. These resources would give children: a healthy start; a safe environment; caring and reliably available adults; an education resulting in

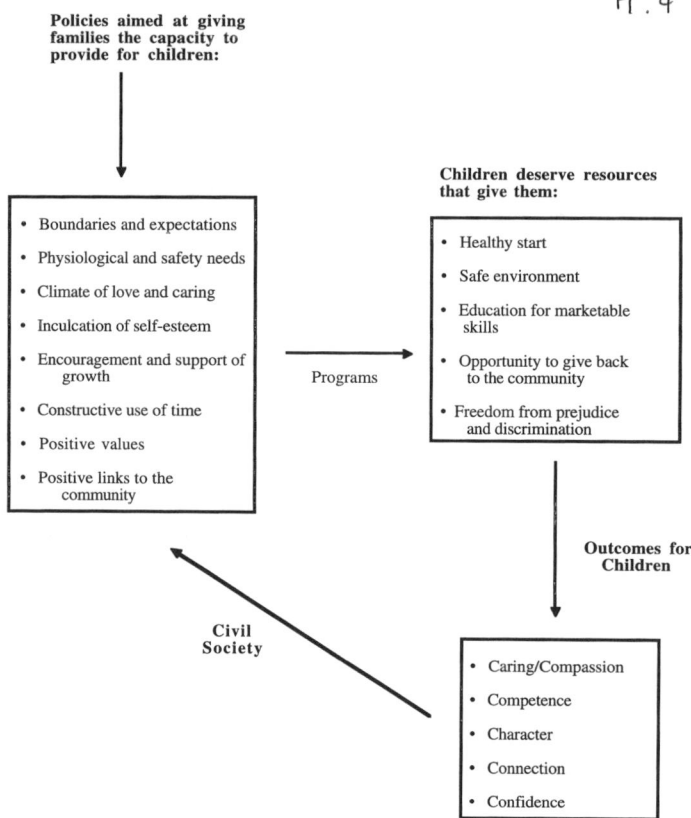

Figure 7.4 *A model of a national youth policy: The integration of families, children, and civil society*

marketable skills; and opportunities to "give back" to their communities—to volunteer and serve.

If programs are effective in delivering such resources several positive developmental outcomes will accrue among children. These outcomes can be summarized by "five Cs:" Competence, Connection, Character, Confidence, and Caring (or Compassion) (Carnegie Council on Adolescent Development, 1989; Lerner, 1995; Little, 1993). These five attributes represent five clusters of individual attributes—for example, intellectual ability and social and behavioral skills; positive bonds with people and institutions; integrity and moral centeredness; positive self-regard, a sense of self-efficacy, and courage; and humane values, empathy, and a sense of social justice, respectively. When these five sets of outcomes are developed, civil society is enhanced.

As indicated in the model displayed in Figure 7.4, such enhancement feeds back to influence the family. The growth of civil society is a resource that facilitates the nurturing and socialization function of families.

Clearly, the key "fuel" to enable such a model for a national youth policy to work is one that builds on the existing assets of communities (e.g., see Figure 4.1).

Family Diversity and Family Policy

These assets are the current "inventory" of civil society in America. Accordingly, these assets need to be employed to build the programs that will be associated with the enactment of the model displayed in Figure 7.4.

IMPLEMENTING THE MODEL: THE POTENTIAL OF COMMUNITY-BASED YOUTH PROGRAMS

How might we develop a system to deliver these assets to youth? Although there are certainly numerous answers to this question, an obvious principle we may use to formulate any answer is to build on the existing assets associated with such delivery. A prominent instance of such an asset is the youth programs that exist in virtually all communities in America.

Whether the community-based programs in a particular community are ones associated with national organizations such as 4-H, the YMCA, Scouting, Little League, or Boys and Girls Clubs, or with the thousands of community-specific, "grassroots" organizations that are present in the communities of our nation, many scholars and advocates for youth believe that it is important to capitalize on the important role played by these youth-serving organizations in attempting to build a system to deliver assets that enhance the life chances of youth (cf. Carnegie Corporation of New York, 1992; Dryfoos, 1990; National Research Council, 1993; Schorr, 1988). Advocates for the support and sustainability of youth-serving programs argue that policies must promote the financial support, and broad acceptance, of community-based youth organizations (Pittman & Zeldin, 1994). Such acceptance involves support of the socialization experiences and youth services provided by these organizations. However, to promote the acceptance of such youth-serving community programs, some advocates argue that "policy goal of facilitating youth development must be translated and incorporated into the public institutions of education, employment and training, juvenile justice, and health services" (Pittman & Zeldin, 1994, p. 53).

Are such policy steps warranted? To answer "yes" to this question requires evidence that youth-serving programs that seek to promote the individual and contextual assets of youth result in positive developmental outcomes. Accordingly, two additional questions are raised: Does evidence that supports a particular set of principles and practices best able to facilitate the healthy development of youth exist? Does the enactment of such "best principles and practices" result in positive developmental outcomes for youth?

COMMUNITY-BASED, POSITIVE YOUTH DEVELOPMENT PROGRAMS: PRINCIPLES AND PRACTICES

The concept of a program specifically designed to enhance the positive development of youth was first introduced into the public policy arena in the late 1960s. However, it was not until 20 years later that the concept became prominent (Roth, et al., 1997). As a result of its relatively short history, there is not complete consensus about the characteristics of such programs (Roth, et al., 1997). Nevertheless, both on an abstract level, in regard to the general principles from which program features should be derived, and on a more concrete level, wherein one compares descriptions of the actual features of programs believed to be effective in the promotion of positive youth development, it is possible to present a coherent depiction of what are regarded to be both "best principles" and "best practices." For instance, Lerner (1995) concluded that the literature about youth development supported at least five generalizations about the challenges facing youth and the implications for programs and policies of these challenges:

1. Youth problem behaviors and poverty are interrelated, and this "comorbidity" is of historic proportions;
2. programs should focus on this interrelation, and on the integration of youth, families, and communities;
3. programs should focus on the assets of individuals and their communities and on strengthening these resources;
4. prevention of problems is not equivalent to the provision of assets for positive development; and
5. policies and programs should seek to promote positive youth development.

Roth, et al. (1997) reached similar conclusions about the principles of effective youth development programs. To illustrate, Roth, et al. (1997) indicated that effective youth programs are predicated on an abiding concern for the well-being of our nation's youth. Such programs transcend traditional intervention (e.g., remediation, alleviation) or prevention strategies; evidence a recognition of the interrelationships among youth problems; and focus on competency building and skill development (and not the prevention of specific problem behaviors), and thus counter risk factors through the enhancement of protective factors. Moreover, caring and civic responsibility are important foci of effective youth programs, and they are assets in the promotion of positive youth development (Benson, 1997). In addition, Roth, et al. (1997) noted that ages 10 to 16 years are the crucial time of transition from childhood to adolescence and should be the age focus of youth development programs.

In addition to this congruence among reviewers about the principles upon which an approach to programs emphasizing positive youth development may be undertaken, there is also a good deal of consensus about the precise features of such programs that are effective in the promotion of positive youth development. In other words, when one attempts to translate within a community the principles of effective youth programming into precise, operationally definable practices, what does one see?

Zeldin (1995, p. 1), writing when he was a member of the Center for Youth Development and Policy Research—an organization founded in 1990 to "create and advance a vision of youth development that specifies not only outcomes by strategies as well,"—asked a similar question: "What are the essential day-to-day experiences that help a young person pass successfully through adolescence into young adulthood and which result in the young person acquiring desirable (positive) behaviors, attitudes, and skills?" Roth, et al. (1997, p. 8) report that the answer of the Center is clear:

> Young people need access to safe places, challenging experiences, and caring people on a daily basis . . . young people need the opportunity for: Challenging and relevant chances for formal and informal instruction and training, including explorations, practice, and reflection as well as expression and creativity; and new roles and responsibilities, including group membership, contribution and service, and part-time paid employment. The support youth need include: ongoing contact with people and social networks who provide emotional support, such as friendships and nurturance; motivational supports such as high expectations, standards and boundaries; and strategic supports, such as options assessment and planning and access to resources.

In turn, Roth, et al. (1997, p. 9) define youth development programs as "intensive, sustained, integrated, inclusive, age-appropriate service delivery systems designed to prepare adolescents for productive adulthood by helping them gain the competencies, knowledge, and sense of self-worth needed to meet the increasing challenges they will face as they mature." They go on to note that effective youth development programs offer social support systems; provide a broad program and sustained services; promote life-skill development; provide the opportunity for community service; and insure the constructive use of time (Roth, et al., 1997).

ARE POSITIVE YOUTH DEVELOPMENT PROGRAMS ACTUALLY EFFECTIVE?

Despite the relatively general agreement about the principles and practices linked to effective youth programs, Roth, et al. (1997) indicate that there are two important issues that suggest that such agreement may be somewhat premature. First, there may be more agreement about what best principles and practices are than there is congruence in the features of the programs actually delivered to youth. Roth, et al. note that there exists an array of approaches to service in programs labeled as ones aimed at serving youth and promoting their positive development. For instance, consistent with the principles and practices deemed best by reviewers of youth-serving programs (e.g., Benson, 1997; Lerner, 1995; Little, 1993; Pittman & Zeldin, 1994; Roth, et al., 1997; Scales & Leffert, 1999; Zeldin, 1995) some programs are characterized by integrated, positive-behavior-focused comprehensive (service and support) approaches. However, other programs take a multibehavioral, but problem-focused (preventive) approach and are not comprehensive in the scope of their services. In turn, there are also single problem-focused non-comprehensive programs and, as well, single component programs with varying goals for adolescent outcomes (Roth, et al., 1997).

In turn, Roth. et al. (1997) note that the evidence is not strong that youth programs—whether they purport to reflect best principles and practices or the precise array of services delivered to youth—actually promote positive developmental outcomes in young people. That is, Roth, et al. (1997) ask if there is empirical evidence to support the view that youth development programs promote positive youth development, especially in youth at-risk for the development of health and behavior problems.

To address this question, Roth, et al. (1997) sought to identify all the youth-serving organizations in the United States and then found all available (published and unpublished) information about whether the programs of these organizations had been evaluated and shown to be effective in the promotion of positive youth development. Roth, et al. found that 500 national youth-serving organizations were listed in *The Directory of American Youth Organizations* (Erickson, 1996). In addition, they found that there were an additional 17,000 not-for-profit organizations in America that classified themselves as youth development agencies.

Roth, et al. (1997) then searched 200 potentially relevant databases for references to programs serving adolescents and found that seven databases proved most relevant: ERIC (4,341 citations), Social SciSearch (609), PsychINFO (504), NCJRS (389), Dissertation Abstracts (208), Mental Health Abstracts (208), and Sociological Abstracts (124). Within these citations, Roth, et al. identified references to prevention and intervention programs for adolescents and extracted publications pertinent to evaluation. They excluded papers that pertained only to program descriptions or to depictions of program curricula. Only 239 references located but—even among these papers—many had to be excluded from consideration as an evidentiary basis for program effectiveness because they did not deal with the empirical evaluation of program outcomes but, instead, presented opinions or editorial-type statements about programs, were book reviews, or reports of measurement development (Roth, et al., 1997). Because of the small pool of references that remained after this culling process, Roth, et al. (1997) sought to find unpublished evaluation studies. As a result they ended up with about 50 evaluation studies of youth-serving programs (Roth, et al., 1997).

However, even among this small pool of studies the quality of the evaluation research evidence was not impressive. Roth, et al. report that many of the nation's oldest and largest youth organizations do not allocate sufficient financial and staff resources for outcome evaluations and, therefore, there are many unsubstantiated claims about the effectiveness of the programs of youth-development organizations. Moreover, in the evaluations that are conducted or that are proposed (e.g., in proposals by youth-serving organizations to funders) there are weak evaluation designs, for instance, involving small sample sizes, poor record keeping, high staff turn-over, and vague program goals (Roth, et al., 1997). In addition, across evaluation studies, Roth, et al. report that there is no clear consensus about the developmental outcomes that should be used to evaluate youth-serving programs and that many evaluation reports fail to include basic demographic information about youth, a description of the methods used to collect or analyze data, or an indication of the empirical bases of conclusions.

Clearly, then, the quality of youth development program evaluation research is deficient in several important ways. On the one hand, it is often not even pursued and, on the other hand, when it is conducted it is fraught with problems of conceptualization, research design, data analysis, and interpretation. The assertion, then, that the application of best principles and practices will result in the promotion of positive youth development is a claim that—unfortunately—is a vast overgeneralization. The magnitude of this overgeneralization may be understood by consideration of the fact that Roth, et al. (1997) were able to find only a few dozen evaluation research studies pertinent to the 17,500 organizations in America whose work constitutes the pool of activities from which one may draw inferences about the effectiveness of youth-serving programs in promoting positive developmental outcomes in young people.

However, all is not completely bleak. Roth, et al. (1997) emphasize that despite the quite limited quantity and quality of the extant evaluation data base, it is possible to extract information about program effectiveness. They conclude that if programs are implemented well, positive youth development can be promoted (Roth, et al., 1997). Moreover, they find that there are three general characteristics of effective programs, and—although we must recognize that the data base about which we are talking must be substantially expanded—there is evidence that these characteristics do reflect the "best principles and practices" ideas described above. Roth, et al. (1997) note that the more features of the "positive youth development" framework possessed by a program, the more likely it was to promote positive youth outcomes. In addition, they indicate that caring adolescent-adult relations are central for program effectiveness, and that program sustainability is related to program effectiveness. Longer-term programs that engage youth across the adolescent years are most effective (Roth, et al., 1997).

There is additional evidence that the confidence placed in the programs offered by youth-serving organizations is warranted. Scales and Leffert (1999) also review the results of evaluations of such youth programs. They find that involvement in effective youth programs is associated with several significant indicators of positive youth development, including increased self-esteem, popularity, sense of personal control, and identity development. In addition, youth in such programs show better development of life skills, leadership skills, decision making skills, and public speaking ability (Scales & Leffert, 1999). Moreover, Scales and Leffert (1999) report that there is an association between participation in effective youth programs, and increased dependability and job responsibility, better communication with family members, fewer instances of problems of loneliness, shyness, and hopelessness, and decreased involvement in risky behaviors such as drug use and juvenile delinquency.

However, Scales and Leffert (1999) also report findings that indicate that not all youth programs result in such positive outcomes for youth. Indeed, many do not. In agreement with Roth, et al. (1997), Scales and Leffert (1999) emphasize that programs that are effective in producing such outcomes are ones that offer a broad array of services and opportunities targeted to the specific needs, interests, and diversity of the youth to which the program is aimed, and offer a supportive setting that promotes good social relationships with peers and program staff. Moreover,

Scales and Leffert (1999) note that effective youth programs collaborate with other activities/organizations available in the community and, in so doing, involve a broad segment of the social ecology of the young person (e.g., his or her family and school). In addition, effective programs involve committed and capable staff who are devoted to the youth in the program, and offer easy access to the services provided by the program. Such programs overcome barriers to participation (e.g., that might arise because of financial or transportation constraints; Scales & Leffert, 1999).

Moreover, Scales and Leffert (1999) agree with Schorr (1988) and Dryfoos (1998) that effective programs also offer intensive and, at the same time, flexible, non-bureaucratic services (to adjust to the diversity of youth participating in them) that are developmentally appropriate and employ staff that are trained in both the features of the program and the diversity of culture and context of the youth participating in it.

It is important to note that both non-governmental organizations (NGOs) and governmental organizations can deliver such community-based positive youth development programs. For example, O'Leary (1998), working from his vantage point as the Secretary of Health and Human Services of the Commonwealth of Massachusetts, describes other characteristics of community-based, but public sector, programs that he has found are effective in serving the needs of youth and families. He indicates that successful programs: minimize duplication of services; integrate state and local services; share information (while protecting confidentiality; build individual and family capacity; are accessible; include program assessments and evaluations; involve joint budgeting and track state and local funding with an eye towards collaboration; and pursues primary prevention/promotion.

Accordingly, youth programs are essential assets in a coordinated effort to promote positive youth development, when they have the characteristics identified by Roth, et al. (1997), Scales and Leffert (1999), and O'Leary (1998) that comprise effective, community-based—and community-wide, integrative, and collaborative (i.e., multi-institutional)—actions. The translation involved in turning such community programs into policy is predicated on the view that the promotion of youth development is not the exclusive province of any single organization or agency, (Dryfoos, 1990; Hamburg, 1992; Schorr, 1988). To the contrary, an integrated, community-wide effort is necessary both to foster positive youth development through such programs (Dryfoos, 1990; Hamburg, 1992; Schorr, 1988) *and* to evaluate the success of these efforts (Weiss & Greene, 1992).

Hamburg (1992) makes a similar point. He suggests three policy initiatives that, together, would enhance the capacity of communities to (a) provide comprehensive and integrated services that (b) promoted positive youth development through (c) the provision of effective programs delivered by a well-trained staff. Thus, Hamburg (1992, p. 166) notes that he would:

> First, use federal and state mechanisms to provide funding to local communities in ways that encourage the provision of coherent, comprehensive services. State and federal funding should provide

incentives to encourage collaboration and should be adaptable to local circumstances.

Second, provide training programs to equip professional staff and managers with the necessary skills. Such programs would include training for collaboration among professionals in health, mental health, education, and social services, and would instill a respectful, sensitive attitude toward working with clients, patients, parents, and students from different backgrounds.

Three, use widespread evaluation to determine what intervention is useful for whom, how funds are being spent, and whether the services are altogether useful.

CONCLUSIONS

Given the evidence that exists about the outcomes of positive youth development programs, it is reasonable to conclude that public policy must move from a focus on just building effective programs to also building cohesive and effective communities (National Research Council, 1993; Pittman & Zeldin, 1994). Indeed, a recent report by the National Research Council (1993) notes that building supportive communities for youth faced with the destruction of their life chances:

> will require a major commitment from federal and state governments and the private sector, including support for housing, transportation, economic development, and the social services required by poor and low-income residents. (p. 239)

Furthermore, Pittman and Zeldin (1994) emphasize that for youth development programs to attain sustained successes across the span of individual lives and multiple generations, issues of individual and economic diversity must be clearly and directly confronted. Specifically, poverty and racism must be a continued, core focus of social policy. We must continue to be vigilant about the pernicious sequelae of poverty among children and adolescents, the vast overrepresentation of minority youth among the ranks of our nation's poor, and the greater probability that minority youth will be involved in the several problem behaviors besetting their generation.

It is clear that the findings of Roth, et al. (1997) and Scales and Leffert (1999) lend support to the idea that there are principles and practices pertinent to positive youth development programs that, if followed, can result in the effective production of valued youth outcomes, especially when effective programs are sustained across adolescence and offer youth a "convoy of social support" (Antonucci, 1989; Kahn & Antonucci, 1980) by caring adults. At the same time, the findings of Roth, et al. (1997) underscore the critical need to incorporate evaluation into the ongoing functioning of all the thousands of youth-serving organizations in America that, currently, give such work little or at best, inadequate, attention. Certainly, we cannot expect funders to support programs that cannot either prove their effectiveness through evaluation or, as well, improve through evaluation the quality of their work and ability to promote positive youth development. We cannot in good conscience try to go to scale with any program unless we are certain that the financial and human resources we are devoting to such expansion are justified by the results of an appropriate evaluation. And we cannot hope to garner the commitment of funders, policy makers, or youth, families, and communities to sustain a program unless we can demonstrate that we are allocating the energies of resources of stakeholders to an effective program. Accordingly, then, issues of program effectiveness, scale, sustainability, and as well concerns about fiscal responsibility and the ethical use of human capital, rest on making sound program evaluation a core part of the activity of all youth-serving programs in America.

Clearly, then, we believe that youth development programs have the potential for promoting positive youth development and that this potential may be actualized when such programs are coupled with sound program evaluation. Accordingly, a youth policy for America should include the procedural requirement that efforts sound program evaluation should be a core component of efforts to link together youth, families, and community-based programs in the service of furthering civil society (see Figure 7.4). Roth, et al. (1997) have congruent recommendations regarding the importance of program evaluation. They suggest that there is a need to evaluate systematically the effectiveness of different programs, especially those directed specifically to diverse youth. Moreover, and consistent with the importance of caring adults in a young person's life (Benson, 1997) and effective youth programs, Roth, et al. (1997) point to the need to ascertain the role of families in youth development programs. Adult family members, as well as other adults in the community, should be inculcated with the knowledge and skills to contribute to youth development programs. Moreover, Roth, et al. note that more attention must be paid to understanding how effective programs may be sustained in communities involved in contributing effectively to youth development programs. Finally, in agreement with the above-noted link between effective, scale, and evaluation, Roth, et al. (1997) point to the importance of learning about program effectiveness before attempting to go to scale.

In sum, the policy recommendations forwarded by Pittman and Zeldin (1994), Hamburg (1992), Roth, et al. (1997), and the National Research Council (1993) stress the importance of comprehensive and integrative actions linking youth, families, programs, evaluation research, and policy makers. These actions involve, then, both proximal community participation and the contributions of broader segments of the public and private sectors; community-based evaluations; diversity; and promoting positive development across the life span.

These views are consistent with those brought to the fore by a developmental contextual perspective. Chapter 8 discusses these ideas.

8 IMPLICATIONS FOR POLICY DESIGN, DELIVERY, AND EVALUATION

From the perspective of developmental contextualism, policies—and the programs that do (or should) derive from them—merge (or, better, synthesize) basic and applied research. They represent the means through which ecologically valid interventions may be enacted. Evaluation of these interventions provides information, then, both about the adequacy of these "applied" endeavors *and* about "basic" theoretical issues of human development—about bases for the enhancement of the life courses of individuals, families, and communities (Lerner & Miller, 1993; Lerner, et al., 1994).

Thus, from the perspective of developmental contextualism, policies, and the evaluation of their influences or outcomes, are actions that allow outreach scholars to make contributions to the understanding of, and to promote service to, the diverse children, adolescents, and families of our nation. However, developmental contextualism provides more than a structure for the integration of basic and applied scholarship; it offers more than a frame for viewing policy engagement and programming as the "methods" for this integration, the enactment of applied developmental science (Fisher & Lerner, 1994). In addition, there are at least six substantive directions for the development of policies pertinent to the youth and families of America that are promoted by developmental contextualism.

The first direction for policy is associated with the fact that developmental contextualism promotes an emphasis on the developmental system (Ford & Lerner, 1992). Within this system, development involves changes in *relations* between the growing person and his or her context (Lerner, 1991). Accordingly, to enhance development and promote positive youth and family development, we must focus our efforts on this system, and not on either the individual (cf. Dryfoos, 1990; Schorr, 1988) or the context per se. As such, policies should be aimed at building programs that enhance *relationships* for youth and families across the breadth of the system, that is, with peers, schools, and indeed across institutions of the proximal community and the more distal society.

Second, we must recognize that the system within which both youth, families, and the programs aimed at them are embedded is also the system that contains the institutions that do (or could) provide resources for the promotion of positive youth and family development. Accordingly, we should use the multiple connections within the developmental system to create innovative approaches to generating resources to design, deliver, evaluate, and sustain effective family- and youth-serving programs.

Little (1993) provides an example of the potential of such innovation. He notes that all too often programs that might have a chance of being effective are not implemented or sustained. Little believes that one of the key reasons for this situation is that the procedure that has been used to secure program funding is not effective. That is, Little (1993) notes that whereas people with ideas start programs, often at a "grass roots" level, they typically have to go to a person with institutional power (e.g., a supervisor or a director/president of an organization) in order to find a potential advocate for the idea of the program. In turn, then, if this person with institutional power is persuaded to be an advocate for the program, he or she would (because of their role) be in a position to approach yet another person, someone with authority over resources (e.g., a program officer of a community foundation), to secure resources for the program. This procedure is, at best, only intermittently successful and, as such, Little (1993) believes it represents a weak link in the system through which program funding occurs. Accordingly, Little (1993) recommends that new linkages be formed in the system between people with influence (i.e., those with control over resources) and people with ideas. For instance, the International Youth Foundation (IYF) promotes direct involvement of program officers from indigenous, grant-making, community foundations with the communities and the programs that they fund. This "systems change" represents an important paradigm shift in the nature of the process involved in funding community-based youth programs.

Along with new linkages, there is also a need for a "meeting of the minds" between community-based programs and the institutions that fund their work. Sparks (1996) discusses the theoretical and ideological mismatch that can occur between these two groups. The staff of community-based programs have an understanding of the problem that is derived from daily interactions with the children and families they serve. They develop perspectives that tend to be more culture-specific and reflective of lived experiences, which often differ with the problem definition resulting from academic research. Funders are more likely to endorse the research-based perspectives because of the position of the academy in the power hierarchy, and to support proposals for funding that reflect this orientation. When program staff develop proposals based on their understanding of the problem, which may disagree with the academic perspective, it is often quite difficult to obtain funding. This can lead to the submission of multiple proposals and result in the receipt of only partial funding.

A third policy implication for youth and family programs that is associated with developmental contextualism also is derived from an understanding of the developmental system within which individuals and families are embedded: A system that is open to change for the better is also open to change for the worse. Accordingly, to effect sustained enhancement of the lives of youth and the functioning of families, we need policies that promote long-term interventions. A one-shot intervention will not "inoculate" a youth or his or her family for life against the potentially risk-actualizing perturbations of the developmental system within which they continue to live. Thus, we need to build (and fund) long-term—

that is, life-span-oriented—"convoys" of social support (Kahn & Antonucci, 1980) in order to reinforce and further the positive developments that may accrue from effective youth and family programs.

The life-span nature of the developmental system within which youth and families are embedded is associated with a fourth implication for the development of policy. Transitions occur across the life-span (Lerner & Spanier, 1980) and, often, these changes are qualitative in nature.

For example, the transitions involved in the period between childhood and early adolescence involve qualitative alterations in thinking abilities (i.e., "formal operational" ability emerges; Piaget, 1950, 1972); emotions and personality (e.g., involving the psychosocial crisis of identity versus role confusions; Erikson, 1959); social relationships (e.g., a shift in primary social group—from parents to peers—occurs; Guerney & Arthur, 1984); and physiology (i.e., a new—sexual—drive and new hormones emerge during this period; A. Freud, 1969; Katchadourian, 1977). Given such qualitative changes, a program that provides a "goodness of fit" (Lerner & Lerner, 1989; Thomas & Chess, 1977) with the characteristics of the person during childhood may not continue to be fit during adolescence. Similarly, a family that is at the beginning stage of the family life cycle (Duvall, 1971) differs qualitatively from one with adolescent children or one wherein the children have left the "nest" and established families of their own. Accordingly, in order to be sure that the features of programs remain qualitatively valid across the life span of individuals and families, we must monitor and calibrate our programs in order to attend to developmental changes and, as well, to contextual transitions (for example, involving the shift from elementary schools to middle or junior high schools; Simmons & Blyth, 1987; or from a family with children to an "empty nest" situation; Duvall, 1971).

A fifth policy implication, one closely related to the idea of transitions across life, pertains to the issue of individual or interfamilial differences (diversity) and of transformations of individuals, families, and their broader contexts. Developmental contextualism stresses that diversity—of individuals, families, contexts (including cultural ones), and individual-context relations—is the "rule" of human behavior and development. "One size," that is, one type of intervention, "does not fit all." Policies and programs that are fit and effective for a family of one social, racial, ethnic, community, or cultural group may be irrelevant, poorly suited, or even damaging to families with other characteristics of diversity. As such, policies and programs must be sensitive to, and organized to provide a goodness of fit with, the pertinent instances of human diversity relevant to the individual, family, or community to which they are directed.

However, it will not be sufficient to just have policies that promote the development of diversity-sensitive programs. Such policies must also promote a continuing awareness that individual differences *increase* as people and families develop across the courses of their life cycles (Baltes, 1987; Duvall, 1971; Lerner & Spanier, 1978; Schaie, 1979). As such, we must enable programs to be adjusted to fit the transformations in the character of individuality of person and family that emerges across life.

For instance, each human, as he or she develops across life, becomes increasingly different from other people as a consequence of his or her individual history of experiences, roles, and relationships (Lerner, 1988; Lerner & Tubman, 1989). Thus, initial characteristics of individuality are continually transformed over the course of life into different instances of individuality. As a consequence of such transformations in individuality, we must develop programs that are attentive to both initial and to emergent characteristics of individuality—of the person, the family and, especially, person-family relations.

The stress on individuality within developmental contextualism leads to a final implication for policy that returns us to the point that the outreach scholarship promoted by this perspective involves a merger of both basic and applied science. Developmental contextualism conceives of evaluation as providing information both about policy and program efficacy and about how the course of human development can be enhanced through policies and programs. Indeed, because the approach to evaluation—that is, development-in-context evaluation (DICE) procedures—promoted by developmental contextualism (Lerner, 1995; Lerner, Ostrom, & Freel, 1995; Ostrom, Lerner, & Freel, 1995) involve the active participation of the individuals served by the program (Weiss & Greene, 1992), evaluation is also a means to empower program participants and to enhance their capacities to engage in actions (i.e., program design, delivery, and evaluation) that promote the positive development of themselves and of their families.

Accordingly, policies should promote the use of participatory-normative evaluation procedures (Weiss & Greene, 1992). Such evaluations will increase understanding of the lives developing within the context of the policies and programs one is implementing *and*, simultaneously, will inculcate greater capacities, and thus further empower the youth, families, and communities involved in the programs that are being evaluated.

The important role that participatory evaluation procedures can play within a developmental contextual approach to youth and family policy raises the issue of the potential contributions of academe and academicians to addressing the problems besetting America's children, families, and communities. If our nation's universities are to be part of effective community coalitions enacting and fostering the continued development of integrative and comprehensive national youth and family policies, social policy innovations must be coupled with alterations in academic policies and practices. Without such changes in the academy, our nation's universities will not be able to be integral participants in addressing the needs of our country's children and families. It is important, then, to discuss some of the changes in the academy's approach to scholarship that may need to be introduced in order for such participation to occur.

A REVISED SCHOLARLY AGENDA

In order to be complete, the integrative research promoted by a developmental contextual view of human development must be synthesized with two other foci. Research in human development that is concerned with one, or even a few, instances

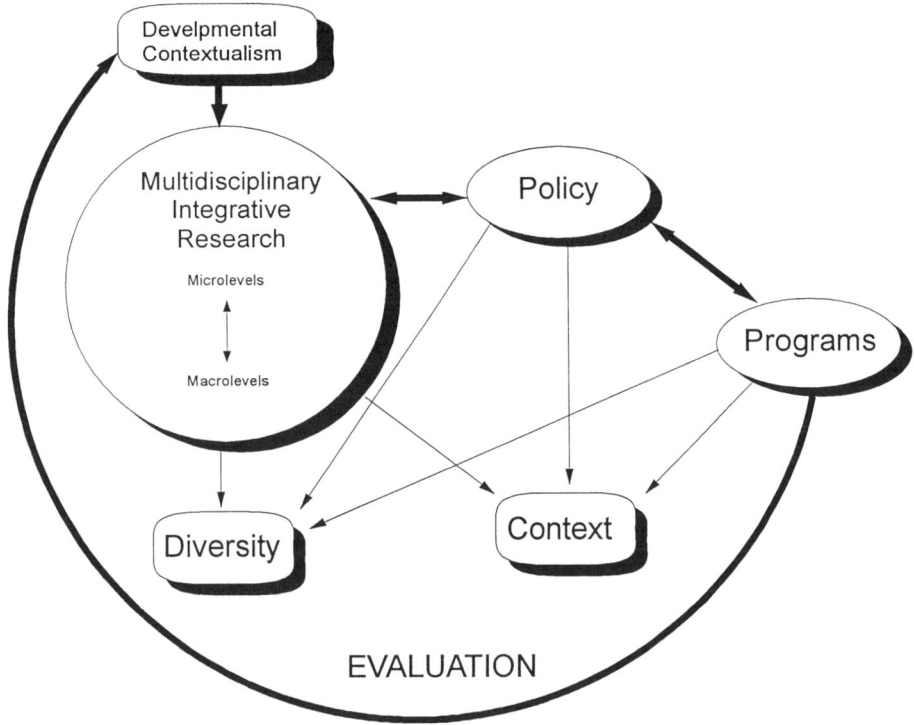

Figure 8.1 *The conception of the integration of multidisciplinary research endeavors centrally aimed at diversity and context, with policies, programs, and evaluation.*

of individual, family, and broader contextual diversity cannot be assumed to be useful for understanding the life course of all people and families. Similarly, policies and programs derived from such research, or associated with it in the context of a researcher's tests of ideas pertinent to human plasticity, cannot be assumed to be applicable, or equally appropriate and useful, for all families or for all individuals. Accordingly, developmental and individual differences-oriented policy development and program (intervention) design and delivery would need to be integrated fully with the new research base for which we are calling (Lerner & Miller, 1993; Lerner, et al., 1994).

As emphasized in developmental contextualism, the variation in settings within which people live means that studying development in a standard (for example, a "controlled") environment does not provide information pertinent to the actual (ecologically valid) developing relations between individually distinct people and their specific contexts (for example, their particular families, schools, or communities). As stressed also in Chapter 3, this point underscores the need to conduct research in real-world settings, and highlights the ideas that: (1) Policies and programs constitute natural experiments, i.e., planned interventions for people and institutions; and (2) the evaluation of such activities becomes a central focus in the developmental contextual scholarly agenda we have described.

In this view, then, policy and program endeavors do *not* constitute secondary work, or derivative applications, conducted after research evidence has been complied. Quite to the contrary, policy development and implementation, and program design and delivery, become integral components of this vision for research; the evaluation component of such policy and intervention work provides critical feedback about the adequacy of the conceptual frame from which this research agenda should derive. This conception of the integration of multidisciplinary research endeavors centrally aimed at diversity and context, with policies, programs, and evaluations is illustrated in Figure 8.1.

Over the past quarter-century, there are been a few scholars who have forwarded a vision of the sort of individual and contextual (or ecological), diversity-sensitive integration of research and policy illustrated in Figure 8.1. Their ideas have framed and continued to frame the policy engagement scholarship of applied developmental scientists. It is useful to discuss the ideas of two of the scholars whose vision has been so influential, Urie Bronfenbrenner and Harriette McAdoo.

THE CONTRIBUTIONS OF BRONFENBRENNER

A vision of the integration between developmental research and policies and programs was articulated more than two decades ago by Bronfenbrenner (1974). Bronfenbrenner argued that engagement with social policy not only enhances developmental research but, consistent with the developmental contextual perspective, it also augments understanding of key theoretical issues pertinent to the nature of person-context relations. Bronfenbrenner (1974) noted that:

> In discussions of the relation between science and social policy, the first axiom, at least among social scientists, is that social policy should be based on science. The proposition not only has logic on its side, but what is more important, it recognizes our proper and primary importance in the scheme of things. The policymakers should look to us, not only for truth, but for wisdom as well. In short, social policy needs science.
> My thesis in this paper is the converse proposition, that, particularly in our field, science needs social policy—needs it not to guide our organizational activities, but to provide us with two elements essential for any scientific endeavor—vitality and validity (p. 1). . . . I contend that the pursuit of [social policy] questions is essential for the further development of knowledge and theory on the process of human development. Why essential? (p. 2). . . . [Because] issues of social policy [serve] as points of departure for the identification of significant theoretical and scientific questions concerning the development of the human organism as a function

of interaction with its enduring environment—both actual and potential. (p. 4)

More than 25 years later, Bronfenbrenner's (1974) ideas about why scholarship needs social policy are illustrated by the key problems he and his colleagues identify as besetting America's children and families (Bronfenbrenner, McClelland, Wethington, Moen, & Ceci, 1996; Bronfenbrenner & Morris, 1998). For instance, Bronfenbrenner, et al. (1996) note that among these problems are the high percentage of youth growing up in single-parent families, the high unemployment rate for parents of young children, the percentage of American children living in poverty, and the growing income disparity between the rich and the poor families of our nation. Reviewing these problems, Bronfenbrenner appeals once again for a science that serves society through its knowledge. He states that:

we have arrived at a point where the concerns of basic developmental science are converging with the most critical problems we face as a nation. That convergence confronts us, both as scientists and as citizens, with new challenges and opportunities. (Bronfenbrenner & Morris, 1998, p. 1022)

The convergence between the key problems facing America's families and children and the need to inform policy makers through research directed to these problems is precisely the emphasis in the ideas of McAdoo (1999). Consistent with the integrative research and application model presented in Figure 8.1, her focus is on the diverse families and children that must garner the attention of policy makers preparing for America of the twenty-first century.

THE CONTRIBUTIONS OF McADOO

McAdoo (1999) proposes six important foci for policy and policy-relevant research pertinent to family diversity, especially given the greatly increasing percentage of the American population that will develop within other than European-American families over the next decades. Included among the recommendations for family policy, and for the scholarship associated with it, is that there should exist:

1. *A focus on culture.* McAdoo indicates that "we need to document children's abilities of coping with stressful situations and the strength of their particular culture. Policies should be examined in light of the group differences that may be problematic for these groups" (McAdoo, 1999, p. 211).

2. *An avoidance of stereotyped and/or non-empirically based views of diverse children and families.* McAdoo (1999, p. 211) notes that research must "explore the wide range of socioeconomic groups that are found in all ethnic groups." Moreover, she emphasizes that when only mean scores are used to represent groups, misleading depictions of both between-group and within-group diversity result.

3. *A sensitivity to the specific country of origin of children and families.* To illustrate this point, McAdoo (1999) criticizes the inclusion of any Spanish-

speaking sample in a group labeled "Hispanic," despite "the very different cultural groups and individual histories that are included" (p. 211) in such a categorization. Similarly, children and families of Chinese, Japanese, Korean, and Vietnamese heritage may be placed in the undifferentiated category "Asian," thus ignoring the different levels of acculturation, contrasting cultural norms, and parenting practices that exist among these groups. McAdoo (1999) cautions researchers that data analyses that fail to ascertain variation associated with such intragroup diversity will involve undue amounts of error variance and will be unable to adequately inform policy.

4. *A willingness to articulate the implications for children of current or to-be-enacted policies.* A key part of the "scholarship of engagement" (Boyer, 1990, 1994), or of "outreach scholarship" (Lerner, 1995, Lerner & Simon, 1998a, 1998b), involves using knowledge to inform policy makers about known or probable associations between social change and human development. Scholars of human development are aware of the import of past and, perhaps, of current policies and programs for healthy youth and family development. Scholars may also extrapolate from the extant literature to make probabilistic statements about the possible influences of policies on young people and their families. We have in fact discussed one instance of such scholarship in Chapter 6, in our presentation of the analysis by Zaslow, et al. (1998) of the relevance of past research on the effects on children of welfare-to-work transition programs to the potential outcomes for children of developing in the current welfare policy context, that is, one framed by the new welfare programs that took effect in 1996 when PRWORA was enacted and signed into law.

This facet of applying developmental science (Fisher & Lerner, 1994; Lerner & Fisher, 1994) is a critical part of the work of scholars involved in the linkage between family diversity and family policy. Indeed, McAdoo (1999) indicates that:

> As researchers it is necessary to respond to new policies that often are not supportive of children. Politics plays a great part in where children and families are today. Family income, welfare, and resources are for the most part politically determined, especially for those of color. As the many changes are occurring in Congress, and in the state capitals of this country, it is often easy to overlook the political realities that are being played out within the lives of families. (p. 212)

5. *A new approach to scholarship, one aimed at engaging community members, including policy makers, must be pursued.* Consistent with a commitment to the scholarship of engagement, researchers must work to expand the range of approaches seen as academically legitimate. In this regard, McAdoo (1999) argues that:

> The usual tactics of conducting studies and simply publishing the results in academic journals is no longer sufficient. Empirical research must provide succinct results. Suggestions of programs of

implementation will have to be specific to the agency or department with which specific policies are related. Issues and monies are moving from the national to the state levels. Researchers had trouble keeping abreast of federal policies, and now it will be necessary to understand up to 50 different state levels of policies of important issues. (p. 214)

The need to engage policy makers in the applied research that is conducted to link the understanding of family diversity to families policies extends to other groups that are invested in the policy making process. More specifically, child- and family-advocacy groups need to be involved in such scholarship. This point leads to a final idea forwarded by McAdoo (1999).

6. *A need for research to be made accessible for advocacy groups.* McAdoo (1999) explains that the scholarship of engagement (outreach scholarship) must involve the translation of research findings into terms understandable to advocacy groups (e.g., the Children's Defense Fund [CDF]), as well as to policy designers (e.g., congressional staff members). Scholars must become capable of offering their work in accessible written and oral formats (e.g., in depositions or in congressional testimony, respectively).

CONCLUSIONS

Both Bronfenbrenner and McAdoo offer visions for the integration of research and policy that serves the needs of the diverse children and families of our nation, and that address the key economic and social disparities that act to diminish social justice and civil society in America. To be successful, their developmental, individual differences, and contextual/ecological views of research, policy, and programs for human development require not only collaboration across disciplines. In addition, the ideas of Bronfenbrenner and of McAdoo indicate that collaboration with both the policy making community and the people whose lives are affected by the policies enacted by policy makers is required. It is useful to discuss these collaborative activities in relation to themes that might organize the future activities of the individuals involved in studying and enhancing human development.

Toward the Creation of an Integrated Agenda for Research and Outreach

As illustrated in Figure 8.1, and as evidenced in the ideas of Bronfenbrenner and of McAdoo, a new research and outreach agenda is brought to the fore by a developmental contextual perspective. This agenda should focus on individual diversity and contextual variation and on the mutual influences between the two. Simply, as we argued in Chapter 3, integrated multidisciplinary and developmental research and outreach devoted to the study of diversity and context must be moved to the fore of scholarly concern.

This integrative research and outreach must be synthesized with two other foci: First, as just discussed, this research must be integrated with policies and programs; and second, this research must involve collaborations among disciplines and between scholarly and community interests.

We have noted both in Chapter 3 and in this chapter that research in human development that is concerned with one or even a few instances of individual and contextual diversity cannot be assumed to be useful for understanding the life course of all people and families. Similarly, policies and programs derived from research insensitive to diversity and context cannot hope to be applicable, or equally appropriate and useful, in all settings or for all individuals or families. Accordingly, developmental and individual differences-oriented policy development and program design and delivery must be key parts of the research base of developmental science. Indeed, when attempts are made to explain the diversity of changing person-context relations that characterizes the human life course, then research-derived outreach (e.g., as depicted in Figure 8.1, program evaluation) becomes a means to test developmental contextual models of change processes.

As we have argued already, because of the variation in settings within which people live, studying development in a controlled environment does not provide information pertinent to the ecologically valid developing relations between individually distinct people and their specific contexts. Predicated, then, on the need to conduct research in real-world settings—and to have the results of such research have meaning to the people in these settings (Bronfenbrenner, 1974; Zigler & Finn-Stevenson, 1992; McAdoo, 1999)—we have suggested that: (a) Policies and programs constitute natural experiments, that is, planned interventions for people and institutions; and (b) the evaluation of such activities becomes a central focus in the developmental systems research agenda we have described (Cairns, 1998; Lerner, 1995; Lerner, Ostrom, & Freel, 1995; Ostrom, Lerner, & Freel, 1995; Zigler & Finn-Stevenson, 1992).

To be successful, this developmental, individual differences, and contextual view of research, policy, and programs for human development requires more than collaboration across disciplines. Multiprofessional collaboration is essential. Colleagues in the research, policy, and intervention communities must plan and implement their activities in a synthesized manner in order to successfully develop and extend this vision. All components of this collaboration must be understood as equally valuable, indeed, as equally essential. The collaborative activities of colleagues in university extension and outreach; program design and delivery; in elementary, middle (or junior high), and high schools; policy development and analysis; and academic research are vital to the success of this new agenda for science and service for children, adolescents, parents, and their contexts, for example, their extended families, schools, workplaces, and communities.

Second, then, given the contextual embeddedness of these synthetic research and outreach activities, collaboration must occur with the people we are trying both to understand and to serve. Without incorporation of the perspective of the community into our work—without the community's sense of ownership, value, and meaning for these endeavors—research and outreach activities cannot be adequately integrated into the lives we are studying.

Thus, from a developmental contextual perspective, research that "parachutes" into the community from the heights of the academy (i.e., that is done in a community without collaboration with the members of the community) is fatally flawed in its ability to understand the process of human development (e.g., see Dryfoos, 1998; Schorr, 1997). This is the case because human development does not happen at the general level (Lerner, 1988, 1991); nor does it occur in a manner necessarily generalizable across diverse people and contexts. Development happens in particular communities, and it involves the attempts of specific children and families to relate to the physical, personal, social, and institutional situations found in their communities. Without bringing the perspective of the community into the "plan" for research, then, the scholar may very likely fail to address the correct problems of human development—the ones involved in the actual lives of the people he or she is studying. And if the wrong problem is being addressed, any "answers" that are found are not likely to be relevant to the actual lives of people. Not surprisingly, these "answers" will be seen all too often (and quite appropriately) as irrelevant by the community.

In turn, however, if the community collaborates in the definition of the problems of development that they and their collaborators are confronting, and if they participate in the construction of the research process, then answers that are obtained will be more likely to be the ones that they wish to know. The answers will be ones more apt to be used to build community-specific policies and programs. Moreover, community empowerment and capacity building occur by engaging in a collaborative process wherein the community places value and meaning on, and participates in, the research and outreach being conducted within its boundaries (Dryfoos, 1990, 1994, 1998; Lerner & Miller, 1993; Lerner, Miller, & Ostrom, 1995; Miller & Lerner, 1994; Schorr, 1988, 1997).

In other words, to enhance ecological validity (or external validity; Hultsch & Hickey, 1978), and provide empowerment and increased capacity among the people we are trying both to understand and serve with our synthetic research and intervention activities, we must work with the community to co-define the nature of our research and program design, and our delivery and evaluation endeavors. In short, we must find ways to apply our scientific expertise to collaborate with, and promote the life chances of, the people participating in our developmental scholarship. Such steps will provide needed vitality for the future progress of the field of human development. As well, however, such steps—by actualizing the integrated agenda for research and outreach for which we are calling—will constitute a paradigm shift in the approach to research pertinent to youth challenged by individual, family, and community risks or stressors.

Paradigm shifts are not easily accomplished in science (Kuhn, 1970). Nevertheless, there is reason to believe that the federal agencies that have traditionally supported research aimed at elucidating means to address youth and family problems are ready to fund the work that will operationalize such a paradigm shift.

From Efficacy- To Outreach-Research

Jensen, Hoagwood, and Trickett (1999) describe two distinct models of research pertinent to the promotion of positive youth development that have been pursued through grants provided by the National Institutes of Health [NIH, e.g., the National Institute of Child Health and Human Development (NICHD) or the National Institute of Mental Health (NIMH)]. The first model—and the one that has been the predominant one in American social and behavioral science—is termed by Jensen, et al. (1999) the "Efficacy Research" model. The key question addressed by research conducted within the frame of this model is: "What works under optimal, university-based, research conditions?"

Studies designed following this model are aimed at determining what is maximally effective under "optimal" (i.e., university-designed, as opposed to "real-world") conditions, in regard to: 1. Preventing the onset of behavioral or emotional problems; 2. ameliorating the course of problems after their onset; and 3. treatment of problems that have reached "clinical" severity. Jensen, et al. (1999) note that the results of the studies conducted within the frame of this model all the conclusion that efficacious preventive interventions for several high risk behaviors and/or outcomes are possible.

However, a second model of research exists—one that has not received the literally hundreds of millions of dollars of NIH support given to efficacy research. Indeed, this second model has been rarely and poorly funded. This second model is one of "outreach" research conducted in "real-world" community settings.

The key question addressed in this model is: "What works that is also: 1. palatable; 2. feasible; 3. durable; 4. affordable; and 5. sustainable in real-world settings?" Jensen, et al. (1999) conclude that when this question is asked then the answer in regard to prevention or positive youth development programs is "Very few (if any), indeed."

Jensen, et al. (1999) argue that the federal government must move, and is in fact now moving, to support outreach research in order to change the answer to the last-noted question to "many, if not most." To create this sea-change in the way scholars conduct their research, Jensen, et al. (1999) recognize that new, more effective partnerships must be created between universities and communities. As we have argued also, Jensen, et al. (1999) believe that there must be a qualitative change in the way universities interact with communities in regard to research pertinent to identifying strategies to promote positive youth development.

Jensen, et al. (1999) argue that such new university-community collaborations should be based on several research-related principles in order to be effective. These principles are consonant with the ideas associated with developmental contextualism and include: 1. an enhanced focus on external validity, on the pertinence of research to the actual ecology of human development (Bronfenbrenner, 1979; Bronfenbrenner & Morris, 1998; Hultsch & Hickey, 1978) as opposed to contrived, albeit well-designed, laboratory-type studies; 2. incorporating the values and needs of community collaborators within research activities; 3. full conceptualization and assessment of outcomes, that is, a commitment to understanding thoroughly both the direct and indirect products of a research-based intervention program on youth and their context and to measuring these outcomes; 4. flexibility to fit local needs and circumstances, that is, an orientation to adjust the design or procedures of the research to the vicissitudes of the community within which the work is enacted; 5. accordingly, a willingness to make modifications to research methods in order to fit the circumstances of the local community; and 6. the embracing long-term perspectives, that is, the commitment of the university to remain in the community for a time period sufficient to see the realization of community-valued developmental goals for its youth.

The principles of "best practice" articulated by Jensen, et al. (1999) may be merged with, or, perhaps better, are built upon—those discussed by Chibucos and Lerner (1999) and Lerner and Simon (1998b). These additional principles include: Co-learning (between two expert systems—the community and the university); humility on the part of the university and its faculty, so that true co-learning and collaboration among equals can occur; and cultural integration, so that both the university and the community can recognize and appreciate each other's perspective.

Moreover, Jensen, et al., differentiate between segments of the community with which the university may collaborate. They describe two community groups with whom such scholarship may be enacted: policy makers and the consumers of (participants in) programs. The challenge is to conduct research that is useful to and used by policy makers and, through the creation of such relevance, to empirically-ground policies for children and adolescents (Jensen, et al., 1999). Such policy engagement scholarship may be directed to several questions: Are current local, state, and federal policies supported by research evidence? Do current local. state, and federal policies run counter to research evidence? And how may research and service funding streams across agencies or public-private groups be merged to study programs and policies already in place, and develop new programs? (Jensen, et al., 1999)

In turn, and consistent with the ideas about collaboration derived from developmental contextualism that were discussed earlier, Jensen, et al. (1999) note that university-community collaborations should occur with the consumers (of programs)—that is, with families (parents and youth), neighborhood leaders, school staff, and community leaders. These are the people who either receive the program or who directly interact with the consumers who are involved in the programs derived from the policies developed by policy makers. Consistent with the principles they articulate about effective principles of university-community collaboration, Jensen, et al. (1999) believe that families (and other consumers) should be active participants in shaping and evaluating programs and that the outreach research framing programs should examine the questions of consumers, not just of researchers. A key intellectual question arising from such outreach scholarship is whether answering consumers' questions increases the ecological (external) validity of the research (Jensen, et al., 1999).

Toward the Building of a Collaborative Nation

The developmental contextual view of the family and, more broadly, of the historical and developmental ecology of individual and family life, helps reduce the incidence of what Elder, et al. (1993, p. 6) term the "blindness to social history and context." Prevalent in much of psychology, and even sociology, it is a blindness which, to paraphrase them (1993, p. 7) has envisioned the child and family as embedded in the atemporal and acontextual realm of abstract developmental theory. This is, to say the least, a curious conceptual stance for a field seemingly focused on change.

A developmental contextual perspective leads us to recognize that if we are to have more than a plausible science of human development, but rather an adequate and sufficient one, we must integratively study individual and familial levels of organization in a relational and temporal manner. Anything less will not constitute adequate science. And if we are to serve America's children and families through our science, and if we are to help develop successful policies and programs through our scholarly efforts, then we must accept nothing less than the integrative temporal and relational model of the child and the family that is embodied in the developmental contextual perspective.

Ultimately, we must all continue to educate ourselves about the best means available to promote enhanced life chances among *all* of our youth and families, but especially those whose potentials for positive contributions to our nation are most in danger of being wasted (Lerner, 1993a, 1993b). The collaborative expertise of the research and program delivery communities can provide much of this information, especially if it is obtained in partnership with strong, empowered communities. Policies promoting such coalitions will be an integral component of a national youth and family development policy aimed at creating caring communities having the capacity to nurture the healthy development of our children and families.

Given the enormous—indeed historically unprecedented—challenges facing the families of America, perhaps especially as they strive to raise healthy and successful children capable of leading our nation productively, responsibly, and morally into the next century (Benson, 1997; Damon, 1997; Lerner, 1995), there is no time to lose in the development of such policies. America as we know it—and, even more, as we believe it can be—will be lost unless we act now. All the strengths and assets of our universities, of all of our institutions, and of all of our people must be marshaled for this effort.

REFERENCES

Abramovitz, M. (1988). *Regulating the lives of women: Social welfare policy from colonial times to the present*. Boston: South End Press.

Adelson, J. (1970). What generation gap? *New York Times Magazine*, 10-45.

Ahlburg, D. A., & De Vita, C. J. (1992). New realities of the American family. *Population Bulletin*, 47(2), 1-44.

Alan Guttmacher Institute. (1994). *Sex and America's teenagers*. New York: Alan Guttmacher Institute.

Allison, K. W. (1993). Adolescents living in "non-family" and alternative settings. In R. M. Lerner (Ed.), *Early adolescence: Perspectives on research, policy, and intervention* (pp. 37-50). Hillsdale, NJ: Erlbaum.

Allison, K. W., & Lerner, R. M. (1993). Integrating research, policy, and programs for adolescents and their families. In R. M. Lerner (Ed.), *Early adolescence: Perspectives on research, policy, and intervention* (pp. 17-23). Hillsdale, NJ: Erlbaum.

Almeida, D. M. & Galambos, N. L. (1991). Examining father involvement and the quality of father-adolescent relations. *Journal of Research on Adolescence*, 1(2), 155-172.

Andrews, J. A., Hops, H., Ary, D. V., & Tildesley, E. (1993). Parental influence on early adolescent substance use: Specific and nonspecific effects. *Journal of Early Adolescence*, 13(3), 285-310.

Annie E. Casey Foundation. (1997). *Kids Count Data Book 1997: State profiles of child well-being*. Baltimore: Annie E. Casey Foundation.

Antonucci, T. C. (1989). Understanding adult social relationships. In K. Kreppner & R. M. Lerner (Eds.), *Family systems and life-span development* (pp. 303-317). Hillsdale, NJ: Erlbaum.

Armistead, L., Wierson, M., & Forehand, R. (1990). Adolescents and maternal employment: Is it harmful for a young adolescent to have an employed mother? Special Issue: Parent work and early adolescent development. *Journal of Early Adolescence*, 10(3), 260-278.

Axinn, J. M., and Hirsch, A. E. (1993). Welfare and the "reform" of women. *Families-in-Society*, 74(9), 563-572.

Baltes, P. B. (1987). Theoretical propositions of life-span developmental psychology: On the dynamics between growth and decline. *Developmental Psychology*, 23, 611-626.

Baltes, P. B., & Baltes, M. M. (1980). Plasticity and variability in psychological aging: Methodological and theoretical issues. In G. E. Gurski (Ed.), *Determining the effects of aging on the central nervous system* (pp. 41-66). Berlin: Schering.

Baltes, P.B., Lindenberger, U., and Staudinger, U. M. (1998). Life-span theory in developmental psychology. In W. Damon (Series Ed.) & R. M. Lerner (Vol. Ed.), *Handbook of child psychology: Vol. 1 Theoretical models of human development* (5th ed., pp. 1029-1143. New York: Wiley.

Baltes, P. B., & Nesselroade, J. R. (1973). The developmental analysis of individual differences on multiple measures. In J. R. Nesselroade & H. W. Reese (Eds.), *Life-span developmental psychology: Introduction to research methodological issues* (pp. 219-251). New York: Academic Press.

Baltes, P. B., Reese, H. W., & Lipsitt, L. P. (1980). Life-span developmental psychology. *Annual Review of Psychology*, 31, 65-110.

Baltes, P. B., Reese, H. W., & Nesselroade, J. R. (1977). *Life-span developmental psychology: Introduction to research methods*. Monterey, CA: Brooks/Cole.

Bane, M. J., & Ellwood, D. T. (1994). *Welfare realities: From rhetoric to reform*. Cambridge, MA: Harvard University Press.

Barber, B.K. (1994). Cultural, family, and person contexts of parent-adolescent conflict. *Journal of Marriage and the Family*, 56, 375-386.

Barnes, G. M., & Farrell, M. P. (1992). Parental support and control as predictors of adolescent drinking, delinquency, and related problem behaviors. *Journal of Marriage and the Family*, 54, 763-776.

Barrera, M., Li, S. A., & Chassin, L. (1995). Effects of parental alcoholism and life stress on Hispanic and non-Hispanic Caucasian adolescents: A prospective study. *American Journal of Psychology*, 23(4), 479-507.

Barringer, F. (1991, March 11). Census shows profound change in racial makeup of the nation. *The New York Times*, pp. 1, A12.

Baumrind, D. (1967). Child care practices anteceding three patterns of the preschool behavior. *Genetic Psychology Monographs, 75,* 43-88.
Baumrind, D. (1971). Current patterns of parental authority. *Developmental Psychology Monographs, 4,* No. 1, Part 2.
Baumrind, D. (1991). The influence of parenting style on adolescent competence and substance use. *Journal of Early Adolescence, 11*(1), 56-95.
Belsky, J., Lerner, R. M., & Spanier, G. B. (1984). *The child in the family.* Reading, MA: Addison-Wesley.
Bennett, N., & Li, J. (1998). *Young child poverty in the states—Wide variation and significant change* (Early childhood poverty research brief 1). New York: National Center for Children in Poverty.
Benson, P. (1997). *All kids are our kids: What communities must do to raise caring and responsible children and adolescents.* San Francisco: Jossey-Bass.
Benson, P. L., Leffert, N., Scales, P. C., & Blyth, D. A. (1998). Beyond the "village" rhetoric: Creating healthy communities for children and adolescents. *Applied Developmental Science,* 2(3), 138-159.
Benson, P. L., & Roehlkepartain, E. C. (1993, June). Single parent families. *Source.* Available from Search Institute, Thresher Square West, Suite 210, 700 South Third Street, Minneapolis, MN 55415.
Bijou, S. W. (1976). *Child development: The basic stage of early childhood.* Englewood Cliffs, NJ: Prentice-Hall.
Bijou, S. W., & Baer, D. M. (Eds.). (1961). *Child development: A systematic and empirical theory.* New York: Appleton-Century-Crofts.
Bijou, S. W., & Baer, D. M. (Eds.). (1965). *Child development: Universal stage of infancy.* Englewood Cliffs, NJ: Prentice-Hall.
Bingham, C. R., & Crockett, L. J. (1996). Longitudinal adjustment patterns of boys and girls experiencing early, middle, and late sexual intercourse. *Developmental Psychology, 32*(4), 647-658.
Birkel, R., Lerner, R. M., & Smyer, M. A. (1989). Applied developmental psychology as an implementation of a life-span view of human development. *Journal of Applied Developmental Psychology, 10,* 425-445.
Blank, H. (1997). Child care in the context of welfare "reform." In S. B. Kamerman & A. F. Kahn (Eds.), *Child care in the context of welfare reform.* (pp.1-44). New York: Cross-National Studies Research Program, Columbia University School of Social Work.
Blum, B. B. (1992). Preface. In S. Smith, S. Blank, & A. Collins, *Pathways to self-sufficiency for two generations: Designing welfare-to-work programs that benefit children and strengthen families.* New York: Foundation for Child Development.
Bogenschneider, K. (1994). *Some thoughts on a two-generational approach in welfare reform.* Available from the School of Family Resources and Consumer Studies, University of Wisconsin, 1430 Linden Drive, Madison, WI 53706-1575.
Bogenschneider, K. (1997). Promoting family-friendly welfare reform: What role can philanthropy play? In K. Bogenschneider, T. Corbett, & M. E. Bell (Eds.), *Welfare reform: Challenges or opportunities for philanthropy? Donor Forum of Wisconsin Briefing Report* (pp. 26-37). Madison, WI: School of Human Ecology, University of Wisconsin-Madison.
Bogenschneider, K., & Corbett, T. (Eds.). (1995). *Welfare reform: Can government promote parental self-sufficiency while ensuring the well-being of children? (2nd ed.). Wisconsin Family Impact Seminars Briefing Report.* Madison, WI: School of Family Resources and Consumer Sciences, University of Wisconsin-Madison.
Bogenschneider, K., Corbett, T., & Bell, M. E. (Eds.). (1997). Welfare reform: Challenges or opportunities for philanthropy? *Donor Forum of Wisconsin Briefing Report.* Madison, WI: School of Human Ecology, University of Wisconsin-Madison.
Bogenschneider, K., Corbett, T., Bell, M. E., & Linney, K. D. (Eds.). (1997). *Moving families out of poverty: Employment, tax, and investment strategies. Wisconsin Family Impact Seminars and The Institute for Research on Poverty Briefing Report.* Madison, WI: School of Human Ecology, University of Wisconsin-Madison.
Bogenschneider, K., Ragsdale, E., & Linney, K. (Eds.). (1995, November). *Child support: the effects of the current system on families. Wisconsin Family Impact Seminars Briefing Report Series.* Available from the School of Family Resources and Consumer Sciences, University of Wisconsin, 1430 Linden Drive, Madison, WI 53706-1575.
Bornstein, M. H. (Ed.). (1995). *Handbook of parenting, Vol. 3: Status and social conditions of parenting.* Mahwah, NJ: Lawrence Erlbaum Associates, Inc.
Bowlby, J. (1969). *Attachment and loss: Vol. 1 Attachment.* New York: Basic Books.
Bowman, H. A., & Spanier, G. B. (1978). *Modern marriage* (8th ed.). New York: Mc-Graw Hill.
Boyer, E. L. (1990). *Scholarship reconsidered: Priorities of the professoriate.* Princeton, NJ: The Carnegie Foundation for the Advancement of Teaching.
Boyer, E. L. (1994, March 9). Creating the new American college. *The Chronicle of Higher Education,* A48.
Brandtstädter, J. (1998). Action perspectives on human development. In W. Damon (Series Ed.) & R. M. Lerner (Vol. Ed.), *Handbook of child psychology: Vol. 1 Theoretical models of human development* (5th ed., pp. 807-863). New York: Wiley.

Bridgman, A., & Philips, D. (Eds.). (1996). *Child care for low income families: Directions for research: Summary of a workshop.* Washington, D.C.: National Academy Press.
Brim, O. G., Jr., & Kagan, J. (Eds.). (1980). *Constancy and change in human development.* Cambridge, MA: Harvard University Press.
Brodkin, K. (1998). *How Jews became whitefolks and what that says about race in America.* New Brunswick, NJ: Rutgers University Press.
Brody, F., & Forehand, R. (1990). Interparental conflict, relationship with the noncustodial father, and adolescent post-divorce adjustment. *Journal of Applied Developmental Psychology, 32*(4), 696-706.
Brody, G. H., Stoneman, Z., & Flor, D. (1996). Parental religiosity, family processes, and youth competence in rural, two-parent African American families. *Developmental Psychology, 32*(4), 696-706.
Bronfenbrenner, U. (1974). Developmental research, public policy, and the ecology of childhood. *Child Development, 45,* 1-5.
Bronfenbrenner, U. (1977). Toward an experimental ecology of human development. *American Psychologist, 32,* 513-531.
Bronfenbrenner, U. (1979). *The ecology of human development.* Cambridge, MA: Harvard University Press.
Bronfenbrenner, U., & Crouter, A. C. (1983). The evolution of environmental models in developmental research. In W. Kessen (Series Ed.) & P.H. Mussen (Vol. Ed.), *Handbook of child psychology: Vol. 1 History, theory, and methods* (4th ed., pp. 357-414). New York: Wiley.
Bronfenbrenner, U., McClelland, P., Wethington, E., Moen, P., &, & Ceci, S. J. (1996). *The state of Americans: This generation and the next.* New York: Free Press.
Bronfenbrenner, U., & Morris, P. (1998). The ecology of developmental processes. In W. Damon (Series Ed.) & R. M. Lerner (Vol. Ed.), *Handbook of child psychology: Vol. 1 Theoretical models of human development* (5th ed., pp. 993-1027). New York: Wiley.
Bronstein, P. Fitzgerald, M., Briones, M., & Pieniadz, J. (1993). Family emotional expressiveness as a predictor of early adolescent social and psychological adjustment. *Journal of Early Adolescence, 13*(4), 448-471.
Brown, B. B., Mounts, N., Lamborn, S. D., & Steinberg, L. (1993). Parenting practices and peer group affiliation in adolescence. *Child Development, 64,* 467-482.
Buchanan, C. M., Maccoby, E., & Dornbusch, S. M. (1991). Caught between parents: Adolescents' experience in divorced homes. *Child Development, 62,* 1008-1029.
Bumpass, L., & Sweet, J. (1989). National estimates of cohabitation. *Demography, 26*(4), 615-625.
Bumpass, L., Raley, R., & Sweet, J. (1994). *The changing character of stepfamilies: Implications of cohabitation and nonmarital childbearing.* Paper presented at Rand Conference, January 20-21, Santa Monica, CA: NSFH Working Paper #63.
Bureau of the Census. (1994). *Supplemental tables, historical income, historical poverty, and valuing non cash benefits.* Washington D.C.: U. S. Department of Commerce.
Burton, L. M. (1990). Teenage childbearing as an alternative life-course strategy in multigeneration black families. *Human Nature, 1*(2), 123-143.
Cairns, R. B. (1998). The making of developmental psychology. In W. Damon (Series Ed.) & R. M. Lerner (Vol. Ed.), *Handbook of child psychology: Vol. 1 Theoretical models of human development* (5th ed., pp. 419-448). New York: Wiley.
Cairns, R. B., & Hood, K. E. (1983). Continuity in social development: A comparative perspective on individual difference prediction. In P. B. Baltes & O. G. Brim, Jr. (Eds.), *Life-span development and behavior* (Vol. 5, pp. 301-358). New York: Academic Press.
Carnegie Corporation of New York. (1992). *A matter of time: Risk and opportunity in the nonschool hours.* New York: Carnegie Corporation of New York.
Carnegie Corporation of New York. (1994, April). *Starting points: Meeting the needs of our youngest children.* New York: Carnegie Corporation of New York.
Carnegie Corporation of New York. (1995). *Great transitions: Preparing adolescents for a new century.* New York: Carnegie Corporation of New York.
Carnegie Council on Adolescent Development. (1989). *Turning points: Preparing American youth for the twenty-first century.* Washington DC: Carnegie Council on Adolescent Development.
Carson, A., Madison, T, & Santrock, J. (1987). Relationships between possible selves and self-reported problems of divorced and intact family adolescents. *Journal of Early Adolescence, 7*(20), 191-204.
Cauce, A. M. (1986). Social networks and social competence: Exploring the effects of early adolescent friendships. *American Journal of Community Psychology, 14,* 607-628.
Cauce, A. M., Felner, R. D., & Primavera, J. (1982). Social support in high-risk adolescents: Structural components and adaptive impact. *American Journal of Community Psychology, 10,* 417-428.
Cauce, A. M., Hannan, K., & Sargeant, M. (1992). Life stress, social support, and locus control during early adolescence: Interactive effects. *American Journal of Community Psychology, 20,* 787-798.
Center for Population Options. (1992). *Teenage pregnancy and too-early childbearing: Public costs, personal consequences.* Washington, DC: Center for Population Options.

Center for the Study of Social Policy. (1992). *1992 Kids Count data book: State profiles of child well-being*. Washington DC: Center for the Study of Social Policy.
Center for the Study of Social Policy. (1993). *Kids Count data book: State profiles of child well-being*. Washington DC: Center for the Study of Social Policy.
Center for the Study of Social Policy. (1995). *Kids count data book*. Washington, DC: Center for the Study of Social Policy.
Chess, S., & Thomas, A. (1984). *The origins and evolution of behavior disorders: Infancy to early adult life*. New York: Brunner/Mazel.
Chibucos, T., & Lerner, R. M. (Eds.). (1999). *Serving children and families through community-university partnerships: Success stories*. Norwell, MA: Kluwer.
Child Welfare League. (1993). *Child Welfare Stat Book 1993*. Washington D. C.: Child Welfare League of America.
Children's Defense Fund. (1992). *Child poverty up nationally and in 33 states*. Washington, DC: Children's Defense Fund.
Children's Defense Fund. (1996). *The state of America's children yearbook*. Washington, DC: Children's Defense Fund.
Chiu, M. L., Feldman, S. S., & Rosenthal, D. A. (1992). The influence of immigration on parental behavior and adolescent distress in Chinese families residing in two western nations. *Journal of Research on Adolescence, 2*, 205-239.
Committee on Ways and Means. (1994). *Overview of entitlement programs*. Washington, D.C.: U.S. Government Printing Office.
Compas, B. E. (1989). Parent and child stress and symptoms: An integrative analysis. *Developmental Psychology, 25*(4), 550-559.
Conger, R. D., Patterson, G. R., & Ge, X. (1995). It takes two to replicate: A mediational model for the impact of parents' stress on adolescent adjustment. *Child Development, 66*, 80-97.
Corbett, T. (1993, Spring). Child poverty and welfare reform: Progress or paralysis? *Focus, 15*(1), 1-17.
Corbett, T. (1995a). Changing the culture of welfare. *Focus, 16*(2), 12-22.
Corbett, T. (1995b). Why welfare is still so hard to reform. In K. Bogenschneider & T. Corbett (Eds.), *Welfare reform: Can government promote parental self-sufficiency while ensuring the well-being of children? (2nd ed.). Wisconsin Family Impact Seminars Briefing Report* (pp. 1-16). Madison, WI: School of Family Resources and Consumer Sciences, University of Wisconsin-Madison.
Corbett, T. (1997). Informing the welfare debate: An overview. In K. Bogenschneider, T. Corbett, & M. E. Bell (Eds.), *Welfare reform: Challenges or opportunities for philanthropy? Donor Forum of Wisconsin Briefing Report* (pp. 7-13). Madison, WI: School of Human Ecology, University of Wisconsin-Madison.
Cost, Quality, and Child Care Outcomes Study Team. (1995). *Cost, quality, and child outcomes in child care centers*. Denver: University of Colorado.
Costa, F. M., Jessor, R., Donovan, J. E., & Fortenberry, J. D. (1995). Early initiation of sexual intercourse: The influence of psychosocial unconventionality. *Journal of Research on Adolescence, 5*, 93-122.
Crystal, D. S., & Stevenson, H. W. (1995). What is a bad kid? Answers of adolescents and their mothers in three cultures. *Journal of Research on Adolescence, 5*(1), 71-91.
Csikszentmihalyi, M., & Rathunde, K. (1998). The development of the person: An experiential perspective on the ontogenesis of psychological complexity. In W. Damon (Series Ed.) & R. M. Lerner (Vol. Ed.), *Handbook of child psychology: Vol. 1 Theoretical models of human development* (5th ed., pp. 635-684). New York: Wiley.
D'Angelo, L. L., Weinberger, D. A., & Feldman, S. S. (1995). Like father, like son? Predicting male adolescents' adjustment from parents' distress and self-restraint. *Developmental Psychology, 31*(6), 883-896.
Damon, W. (1997). *Youth charter: How communities can work together to raise standards for all our children*. New York: The Free Press.
Darwin, C. (1872). *The expression of emotion in men and animals*. London: J. Murray.
Davidson, C. E. (1994). Dependent children and their families: A historical survey of United States policies. In F. H. Jacobs & M. W. Davies (Eds.), *More than kissing babies? Current child and family policy in the Unites States* (pp. 65-89). Westport, CT: Auburn House.
Davies, M. W., & Jacobs, F. H. (1994). Considering race, class, and gender in child and family policy. In F. H. Jacobs & M. W. Davies (Eds.), *More than kissing babies? Current child and family policy in the Unites States* (pp. 265-276). Westport, CT: Auburn House.
Demo, D.H., & Acock, A.C. (1988). The impact of divorce on children. *Journal of Marriage and the Family, 50*, 619-648.
di Mauro, D. (1995). *Sexuality research in the United States: An assessment of social and behavioral sciences*. New York: The Social Science Research Council.
Dixon, R. A., & Lerner, R. M. (1999). History and systems in developmental psychology. In M. Bornstein & M. Lamb (Eds.), *Developmental psychology: An advanced textbook* (4th ed., pp. 3-45). Mahwah, NJ: Erlbaum.
Doherty, W. J., & Needle, R. H. (1991). Psychological adjustment and substance use among adolescents before and after a parental divorce. *Child Development, 62*, 328-337.

Dryfoos, J. G. (1990). *Adolescents at risk: Prevalence and prevention.* New York: Oxford University.
Dryfoos, J. G. (1994). *Full service schools: A revolution in health and social services of children, youth and families.* San Francisco: Jossey-Bass.
Dryfoos, J. G. (1998). *Safe passage: Making it through adolescence in a risky society.* New York: Oxford University Press.
Dubois, D. L., Eitel, S. K., & Felner, R. D. (1994). Effects of family environment and parent-child relationships on school adjustment during the transition to early adolescence. *Journal of Marriage and the Family, 56,* 405-414.
Duncan, G. J. (1991). The economic environment of childhood. In A. C. Huston (Ed.), *Children in poverty: Child development and public policy* (pp. 23-50). Cambridge: Cambridge University.
Duncan, G. D., Hill, M. S., & Hoffman, S. D. (1988). Welfare dependence within and across generations. *Science, 239,* 467-471.
Durbin, D. L., Darling, N., Steinberg, L., & Brown, B. B. (1993). Parenting style and peer group membership among European-American adolescents. *Journal of Research on Adolescence, 3*(1), 87-100.
Duvall, E. M. (1971). *Family development* (4th ed.). Philadelphia, PA: J.P. Lippincott.
East, P. L. (1989). Early adolescents' perceived interpersonal risks and benefits: Relations to social support and psychological functioning. *Journal of Early Adolescence, 2*(4), 374-395.
East, P. L., Felice, M. E., & Morgan, M. C. (1993). Sisters' and girlfriends' sexual and childbearing behavior: Effects on early adolescent girls' sexual outcomes. *Journal of Marriage and the Family, 55,* 953-963.
Eisenberg, N., & McNally, S. (1993). Socialization and mothers' and adolescents' empathy-related characteristics. *Journal of Research on Adolescence, 3*(2), 171-191.
Elder, G. H., Jr. (1974). *Children of the Great Depression: Social change in life experiences.* Chicago: University of Chicago Press.
Elder, G. H., Jr. (1980). Adolescence in historical perspective. In J. Adelson (Ed.), *Handbooks of adolescent psychology* (pp. 3-46). New York: Wiley.
Elder, G. H., Jr. (1998). The life course and human development. In W. Damon (Series Ed.) & R. M. Lerner (Vol. Ed.), *Handbook of child psychology: Vol. 1 Theoretical models of human development* (5th ed., pp. 939-991). New York: Wiley.
Elder, G. H., Jr., Modell, J., & Parke, R. D. (Eds.). (1993). *Children in time and place: Developmental and historical insights.* New York: Cambridge University Press.
Erickson, J. B. (1996). *Directory of American youth organizations 1996-1997.* Minneapolis, MN: Free Spirit Publishing.
Erikson, E. H. (1959). Identity and the life-cycle. *Psychological Issues, 1,* 18-164.
Featherman, D. L., & Lerner, R. M. (1985). Ontogenesis and sociogenesis: Problematics for theory about development across the lifespan. *American Sociological Review, 50,* 659-676.
Featherman, D. L., Spenner, K. I., & Tsunematsu, N. (1988). Class and the socialization of children: Constancy, change, or irrelevance? In R. M. Lerner, E. M. Hetherington, & M. Perlmutter (Eds.), *Child development in life-span perspective* (pp. 67-90). Hillsdale, NJ: Erlbaum.
Feldman, S. S., Mont-Reynaud, R., & Rosenthal, D. A. (1992). When east moves west: The acculturation of values of Chinese adolescents in the U.S. and Australia. *Journal of Research on Adolescence, 2*(2), 147-173.
Feldman, S. S., Rosenthal, D. R., Brown, N. L., & Canning, R. D. (1995). Predicting sexual experience in adolescent boys from peer rejection and acceptance during childhood. *Journal of Research on Adolescence, 5*(4), 387-412.
Feldman, S. S., & Weinberger, D. A. (1994). Self-restraint as a mediator of family influences on boys' delinquent behavior: A longitudinal study. *Child Development, 65,* 195-211.
Feldman, S. S., & Wood, D.N. (1994). Parents' expectations for preadolescent sons' behavioral autonomy: A longitudinal study of correlates and outcomes. *Journal of Research on Adolescence, 4*(1), 45-70.
Felner, R. D., Aber, M. S., Primavera, J., & Cauce, A. M. (1985). Adaptation and vulnerability in high-risk adolescents: An examination of environmental mediators. *American Journal of Community Psychology, 13,* 365-379.
Fine, M. A., & Kurdek, L. A. (1992). The adjustment of adolescents in stepfather and stepmother families. *Journal of Marriage and the Family, 54,* 725-736.
Finkelstein, J. W. (1993). Familial influences on adolescent health. In R. M. Lerner (Ed.), *Early adolescence: Perspectives on research, policy and intervention* (pp. 111-126). Hillsdale, NJ: Erlbaum.
Fisher, C. B., & Brennan, M. (1992). Application and ethics in developmental psychology. In D. L. Featherman, R. M. Lerner, & M. Perlmutter (Eds.), *Life-span development and behavior* (Vol. 11, pp. 189-219). Hillsdale, N. J.: Erlbaum.
Fisher, C. B., Jackson, J. F., & Villarruel, F. A. (1998). The study of African American and Latin American children and youth. In W. Damon (Series Ed.) and R. M. Lerner (Vol. Ed.), *Handbook of child psychology: Vol. 1 Theoretical models of human development* (5th ed., pp. 1145-1207). New York: Wiley.
Fisher, C.B. & Johnson, B.L. (1990). Getting mad at mom and dad: Children's changing views of family conflict. *International Journal of Behavioral Development, 13*(1), 31-48.

Fisher, C. B., & Lerner, R. M. (Eds.). (1994). *Applied developmental psychology.* New York: McGraw-Hill.
Fisher, C. B., & Tryon, W. W. (1990). Emerging ethical issues in an emerging field. In C. B. Fisher & W. W. Tryon (Eds.), *Ethics in applied developmental psychology: Emerging issues in an emerging field* (pp. 1-15). Norwood, NJ: Ablex.
Flanagan, C.A., & Eccles, J.S. (1993). Changes in parents' work status and adolescents' adjustment at school. *Child Development, 64,* 246-257.
Ford, D. L., & Lerner, R. M. (1992). *Developmental systems theory: An integrative approach.* Newbury Park, CA: Sage.
Freedman, D. G. (1979). *Human sociobiology: A holistic approach.* New York: Free Press.
Freedman-Doan, C. R., Arbreton, A. J., Harold, R. D., & Eccles, J. S. (1993). Looking forward to adolescence: Mothers' and fathers' expectations for affective and behavioral change. *Journal of Early Adolescence, 13*(4), 472-502.
Freud, A. (1969). Adolescence as a developmental disturbance. In G. Caplan & S. Lebovier (Eds.), *Adolescence* (pp. 5-10). New York: Basic Books.
Freud, S. (1949). *Outline of psychoanalysis.* New York: Norton.
Freud, S. (1954). *Collected works.* London: Hogarth.
Furstenberg, F. F., Jr., & Cherlin, A. J. (1991). *Divided families: What happens to children when parents part.* Cambridge, MA: Harvard University Press.
Galambos, N. L., & Almeida, D. M. (1992). Does parent-adolescent conflict increase in early adolescence? *Journal of Marriage and the Family, 54,* 737-747.
Galambos, N. L., & Maggs, J. L. (1990). Putting mothers' work-related stress in perspective: Mothers and adolescents in dual-earner families. *Journal of Early Adolescence, 10*(3), 313-328.
Galambos, N. L., & Maggs, J. L. (1991). Out-of-school care of young adolescents and self-reported behavior. *Developmental Psychology, 27*(4), 644-655.
Galambos, N. L., Sears, H. A., Almeida, D. M., & Kolaric, G. C. (1995). Parents' work overload and problem behavior in young adolescent. *Journal of Research on Adolescence, 5*(2), 201-223.
Gallimore, M., & Kurdek, L. A. (1992). Parent depression and parent authoritative discipline as correlates of young adolescents' depression. *Journal of Early Adolescence, 12*(2), 187-196.
Garbarino, J. (1992). *Children and families in the social environment* (2nd ed.). New York: Aldine de Gruyter.
García Coll, C., Lamberty, G., Jenkins, R., McAdoo, H. P., Crnic, K., Wasik, B. H., & Vázquez García, H. (1996). An integrative model for the study of developmental competencies in minority children. *Child Development, 67,* 1891-1914.
Garfinkel, I., & McLanahan, S. (1986). *Single mothers and their children: A new American dilemma.* Washington, DC: Urban Institute Press.
Garfinkel, I., & McLanahan, S. (1994). Single mother families and government policy. In S. H. Danziger, G. D. Sandefur, & D. H. Weinberg (Eds.), *Confronting poverty: Prescriptions for change.* Cambridge, MA: Harvard University Press.
Ge, X., Best, K. M., Conger, R. D., & Simons, R. L. (1996). Parenting behaviors and the occurence and co-occurence of adolescent depressive symptoms and conduct problems. *Developmental Psychology, 32*(4), 717-731.
Geertz, C. (1963). The integrative revolution. In C. Geertz (Ed.), *Old societies and new states: The quest for modernity in Asia and Africa* (pp. 105-157). Glencoe, IL: Free Press.
Gewirtz, J. L., & Stingle, K. G. (1968). Learning of generalized imitation as the basis for identification. *Psychological Review, 75,* 374-397.
Gjerde, P. F., & Shimizu, H. (1995). Family relationships and adolescent development in Japan: A family-systems perspective on the Japanese family. *Journal of Research on Adolescence, 5*(3), 281-318.
Gollin, E. S. (1981). Development and plasticity. In E. S. Gollin (Ed.), *Developmental plasticity: Behavioral and biological aspects of variations in development* (pp. 231-251). New York: Academic Press.
Gottlieb, G. (1992). *Individual development and evolution: The genesis of novel behavior.* New York: Oxford University Press.
Gottlieb, G. (1997). *Synthesizing nature-nurture: Prenatal roots of instinctive behavior.* Mahwah, NJ: Erlbaum.
Gottschalk, P., McLanahan, S., & Sandefur, G. D. (1994). The dynamics and intergenerational transmission of poverty and welfare participation. In S. H. Danziger, G. D. Sandefur & D. H. Weinberg (Eds.), *Confronting poverty: Prescriptions for change* (pp. 85-108). Cambridge, MA: Harvard University Press.
Gould, S. J. (1977). *Ontogeny and phylogeny.* Cambridge: Belknap Press of Harvard.
Greenberger, E., & Chen, C. (1996). Perceived family relationships and depressed mood in early and late adolescence: A comparison of European and Asian Americans. *Developmental Psychology, 32*(4), 707-716.
Guerney, L., & Arthur, J. (1984). Adolescent social relationships. In R. M. Lerner & N. L. Galambos (Eds.), *Experiencing adolescents: A sourcebook for parents, teachers, and teens.* New York: Garland.

Hagen, J. W., Paul, B., Gibb, S., & Wolters, C. (1990, March). Trends in research as reflected by publications in *Child Development*: 1930-1989. In *Biennial Meeting of the Society for Research on Adolescence*. Atlanta, GA.
Hahn, A. B. (1994). Towards a national youth development policy for young African-American males: The choices policymakers face. In R. B. Mincy (Ed.), *Nurturing young black males: Challenges to agencies, programs, and social policy* (pp. 165-186). Washington, DC: The Urban Institute Press.
Hamburg, D. A. (1992). *Today's children: Creating a future for a generation in crisis*. New York: Time Books.
Harris, I. B. (1994). *Should public policy be concerned with early childhood development?* Harris Graduate School of Public Policy Studies, The University of Chicago, 1155 East 60th Street, Chicago, IL 60637.
Hartup, W. W. (1978). Perspectives on child and family interactions: Past, present, and future. In R. M. Lerner & G. B. Spanier (Eds.), *Child influences on marital and family interaction: A life-span perspective* (pp. 23-45). New York: Academic Press.
Hayes, C.D. (Ed.). (1987). *Risking the future: Adolescent sexuality, pregnancy, and childbearing*. Washington, D.C.: National Academy Press.
Hebb, D. O. (1970). A return to Jensen and his social critics. *American Psychologist, 25*, 568.
Heller, S. (1999, January 29). The several roads to respectability: Scholars examine how Jews fit into America. *The Chronicle of Higher Education, XLV*, A23.
Henry, W. (1990, April 9). Beyond the melting pot. *Time*, p. 28-31.
Hernandez, D. J. (1993). *America's children: Resources from family, government, and the economy*. New York: Russell Sage Foundation.
Hernandez, D. J. (1994). Children's changing access to resources: A historical perspective. *Social Policy Report,8*(1), 1-21.
Hetherington, E. M. (1991). Presidential address: Families, lies, and videotapes. *Journal of Research on Adolescence, 1*, 323-348.
Hetherington, E.M. (1993). An overview of the Virginia longitudinal study of divorce and remarriage with a focus on early adolescence. *Journal of Family Psychology, 7*, 39-56.
Hetherington, E.M., Cox, M., & Cox, R. (1985). Long-term effects of divorce and remarriage on the adjustment of children. *Journal of the American Academy of Child Psychiatry,24*, 815-830.
Hirsch, J. (1970). Behavior-genetic analysis and its biosocial consequences. *Seminars in Psychiatry, 2*, 89-105.
Hofferth, S. L. (1995). Caring for children at the poverty line. *Children and Youth Services Review, 17*(1/2), 1-21.
Hoffman, R. F. (1978). Developmental changes in human infant visual-evoked potentials to patterned stimuli recorded at different scalp locations. *Child Development, 49*, 110-118.
Hogan, R., Johnson, J. A., & Emler, N. P. (1978). A socioanalytic theory of moral development. *New Directions for Child Development, 2*, 1-18.
Holmbeck, G. N., & Hill, J. P. (1991). Conflictive engagement, positive affect, and menarche in families with seventh-grade girls. *Child Development, 62*, 1030-1048.
Homans, G. C. (1961). *Social behavior: Its elementary forms*. New York: Harcourt, Brace, & World.
Howard, J. (1978). The influence of children's developmental dysfunction on marital quality and family interaction. In R. M. Lerner & G. B. Spanier (Eds.), *Child influences on marital and family interaction: A life-span perspectives* (pp. 275-298). New York: Academic Press.
Howes, C. & Smith, E. (1994). *Effects of typical child care on children in poverty*. Paper presented at research briefing, Board on Children and Families, December 5-6, 1994. Los Angeles: University of California
Hultsch, D. F., & Hickey, T. (1978). External validity in the study of human development: Theoretical and methodological issues. *Human Development, 21*, 76-91.
Hunt, E., Streissguth, A. P., Kerr, B., & Olson, H. C. (1995). Mothers' alcohol consumption during pregnancy: Effects on spatial-visual reasoning in 14-year-old children. *Psychological Society, 6* (339-342).
Huston, A. C. (Ed.). (1991). *Children in poverty: Child development and public policy*. Cambridge: Cambridge University Press.
Indian Health Services. (1995). *Trends in Indian Health--1995 Tables*. Rockville, MD: Division of Program Statistics, Office of Planning, Evaluation, and Legislation, Public Health Service, Department of Health and Human Services.
Ignatiev, N. (1995). *How the Irish became white*. New York: Routledge.
Itzkovitz, D. (1998). Passing like me. *South Atlantic Quarterly, Fall*.
Jacobs, F. H. (1994). Child and family policy: Framing the issues. In F. H. Jacobs & M. W. Davies (Eds.), *More than kissing babies? Current child and family policy in the United States* (pp. 9-35). Westport, CT: Auburn House.
Jacobs, F. H., & Davies, M. W. (Eds.). (1994). *More than kissing babies? Current child and family policy in the Unites States*. Westport, CT: Auburn House.
Jacobson, M. F. (1998). *Whiteness of a different color: European immigrants and the alchemy of race*. Cambridge, MA: Harvard University Press.

Jacobvitz, D.B., & Bush, N.F. (1996). Reconstructions of family relationships: Parent-child alliances, personal distress, and self-esteem. *Developmental Psychology, 32*(4), 732-743.

Jensen, P. S., Hoagwood, K., & Trickett, E. (1999). Ivory towers or earthen trenches?: Community collaborations to foster "real world" research. *Applied Developmental Science, 3*(4), 206-212.

Joebgen, A. M., & Richards, M. H. (1990). Maternal education and employment: Mediating maternal and adolescent emotional adjustment. *Journal of Early Adolescence, 10*(3), 329-343.

Johanson, D. C., & Edey, M. A. (1981). *Lucy: The beginnings of humankind*. New York: Simon & Schuster.

Kahn, R. L., & Antonucci, T. C. (1980). Convoys over the life course: Attachment, roles, and social support. In P. B. Baltes & O. G. Brim (Eds.), *Life-span development and behavior, 3* (pp. 253-286). Hillsdale, NJ: Erlbaum.

Kamerman, S., & Kahn, A. (Eds.). (1978). *Family policy: Government and families in fourteen countries*. New York: Columbia University Press.

Kandel, D. B., Rosenbaum, E., & Chen, K. (1994). Impact of maternal drug use and life experiences on preadolescent children born to teenage mothers. *Journal of Marriage and the Family, 56*, 325-340.

Kandel, D. B., & Wu, P. (1995). The contributions of mothers and fathers to the intergenerational transmission of cigarette smoking and adolescence. *Journal of Research on Adolescence, 5*(2), 225-252.

Katchadourian, H. (1977). *The biology of adolescence*. San Francisco: Freeman.

Keith, J., Nelson, C., Schlabach, J., & Thompson, C. J. (1990). The relationship between parental employment and three measures of early adolescent responsibility: Family-related, personal, and social. *Journal of Early Adolescence,10*(3), 399-415.

Kendall, P. C., Chansky, T. E., & Kortlander, E. (1994). Childhood interventions. In R. M. Lerner & C. B. Fisher (Eds.), *Applied developmental psychology* (pp. 407-434). New York: McGraw-Hill.

Kenny, M. E., Moilanen, D. L., Lomax, R., & Brabeck, M. M. (1993). Contributions of parental attachments to view of self and depressive symptoms among early adolescents. *Journal of Early Adolescence, 13*(4), 408-430.

Klerman, L. V. (1991). The health of poor children: Problems and programs. In A. C. Huston (Ed.), *Children in poverty: Child development and public policy* (pp. 1-22). Cambridge: Cambridge University.

Knight, B.P., Virdin, L.M., & Roosa, M. (1994). Socialization and family correlates of mental health outcomes among Hispanic and Anglo American children: Consideration of cross-ethnic scalar equivalence. *Child Development,65*, 212-224.

Kondratas, A. (1997). Reflections on national welfare policy and state reform options. In K. Bogenschneider, T. Corbett, & M. E. Bell (Eds.), *Welfare reform: Challenges or opportunities for philanthropy? Donor Forum of Wisconsin Briefing Report* (pp. 1-6). Madison, WI: School of Human Ecology, University of Wisconsin-Madison.

Kossek, E. E., Huber-Yoder, M., Castellino, D., & Lerner, J. V. (1997). The working poor: Locked out of careers and the organizational mainstream. *Academy of Management Special Issue--Career in the Twenty-first Century, 11*, 75-90.

Krampen, G. (1989). Perceived childrearing practices and the development of locus of control in early adolescence. *International Journal of Behavioral Development, 12*, 177-193.

Kretzmann, J. P., & McKnight, J. L. (1993). *Building communities from the inside out: A path toward finding and mobilizing a community's assets*. Available from Center for Urban Affairs and Policy Research, Northwestern University, 2040 Sheridan Road, Evanston, IL 60208.

Kuhn, T. S. (1970). *The structure of scientific revolutions* (2nd ed.). Chicago: University of Chicago Press.

Lamborn, S. D., Mounts, N. S., Steinberg, L., & Dornbusch, S. M. (1991). Patterns of competence and adjustment among adolescents from authoritative, authoritarian, indulgent, and neglectful families. *Child Development, 62*, 1049-1065.

Larson, R. W., & Richards, M. H. (1994). Family emotions: Do young adolescents and their parents experience the same states? *Journal of Research on Adolescence, 4*(4), 567-583.

Lee, V. E., Burkam, D. T., Zimiles, H., & Ladewski, B. (1994). Family structure and its effect on behavioral and emotional problems in young adolescents. *Journal of Research on Adolescence, 4*(3), 405-437.

Leffert, N., Benson, P. L., Scales, P. C., Sharma, A. R., Drake, D. R., & Blyth, D. A. (1998). Developmental assets: Measurement and prediction of risk behaviors among adolescents. *Applied Developmental Science, 2*(4), 209-330.

Lerner, J. V. (1994). *Working women and their families*. Thousand Oaks, CA: Sage.

Lerner, J. V. & Galambos, N. L. (1985). Mother role satisfaction, mother-child interaction, and child temperament: A process model. *Developmental Psychology,21*(6), 1157-1164.

Lerner, J.V. & Galambos, N. L. (Eds.). (1991). *Employed mothers and their children*. New York: Garland Publishing.

Lerner, J. V., & Lerner, R. M. (1983). Temperament and adaptation across life: Theoretical and empirical issues. In P. B. Baltes & O. G. Brim, Jr. (Eds.), *Life-span development and behavior* (Vol. 5., pp. 197-230). New York: Academic Press.

Lerner, R. M. (1978). Nature, nurture, and dynamic interactionism. *Human Development, 21*, 1-20.

Lerner, R. M. (1979). A dynamic interactional concept of individual and social relationship development. In R. L. Burgess & T. L. Huston (Eds.), *Social exchange in developing relationships* (pp. 271-305). New York: Academic.
Lerner, R. M. (1982). Children and adolescents as producers of their own development. *Developmental Review, 2,* 342-370.
Lerner, R. M. (1984). *On the nature of human plasticity.* New York: Cambridge University.
Lerner, R. M. (1986). *Concepts and theories of human development* (2nd ed.) New York: Random House.
Lerner, R. M. (1987). A life-span perspective for early adolescence. In R. M. Lerner & T. T. Foch (Eds.), *Biological-psychosocial interactions in early adolescence* (pp. 9-34). Hillsdale, NJ: Erlbaum.
Lerner, R. M. (1988). Early adolescent transitions: The lore and laws of adolescence. In M. D. Levine & E. R. McArarney (Eds.), *Early adolescent transitions* (pp. 1-21). Lexington, MA: D. C. Heath.
Lerner, R. M. (1991). Changing organism-context relations as the basic process of development: A developmental-contextual perspective. *Developmental Psychology,27,* 27-32.
Lerner, R. M. (1992). Diversity. *SRCD Newsletter,* pp. 2, 12.
Lerner, R. M. (1993a). Investment in youth: The role of home economics in enhancing the life chances of America's children. *AHEA Monograph Series, 1,* 5-34.
Lerner, R. M. (1993b). Early adolescence: Toward an agenda for the integration of research, policy, and intervention. In R. M. Lerner (Ed.), *Early adolescence: Perspectives on research, policy, and intervention* (pp. 1-13). Hillsdale, NJ: Erlbaum.
Lerner, R. M. (1995). *America's youth in crisis: Challenges and options for programs and policies.* Thousand Oaks, CA: Sage.
Lerner, R. M. (1996). Relative plasticity, integration, temporality, and diversity in human development: A developmental contextual perspective about theory, process, and method. *Developmental Psychology, 32*(4), 781-786.
Lerner, R. M. (Ed.). (1998a). *Theoretical models of human development.* Volume 1 of the *Handbook of child psychology* (5th ed.). Editor-in-Chief: William Damon. New York: Wiley.
Lerner, R. M. (1998b). Theories of human development: Contemporary perspectives. In W. Damon (Series Ed.) & R. M. Lerner (Vol. Ed.), *Handbook of child psychology: Vol 1 Theoretical models of human development* (5th ed., pp. 1-24). New York: Wiley.
Lerner, R. M., Bogenschneider, K., Wilcox, B., Fitzsimmons, E., & Hoopfer, L. C. (1995, February). *Welfare reform and the role of Extension programming* (prepared for the North Central Extension Directors). Available from the Institute for Children, Youth, and Families, Suite 27 Kellogg Center, Michigan State University, East Lansing, MI 48824.
Lerner, R. M., & Busch-Rossnagel, N. A. (Eds.). (1981). *Individuals as producers of their development: A life-span perspective.* New York: Academic Press.
Lerner, R. M., Castellino, D. R., Terry, P. A., Villarruel, F. A., & McKinney, M. H. (1995). A developmental contextual perspective on parenting. In M. H. Bornstein (Ed.), *Handbook of parenting: Vol. II. Biology and ecology of parenting* (pp. 285-309). Hillsdale, NJ: Erlbaum.
Lerner, R. M., & Galambos, N. L. (1998). Adolescent development: Challenges and opportunities for research, programs, and policies. In J. T. Spence (Ed.), *Annual Review of Psychology* (Vol. 49, pp. 413-446). Palo Alto, CA: Annual Reviews.
Lerner, R. M., & Hood, K. E. (1986). Plasticity in development: Concepts and issues for intervention. *Journal of Applied Developmental Psychology, 7,* 139-152.
Lerner, R. M., & Fisher, C. B. (1994). From applied developmental psychology to applied developmental science: Community coalitions and collaborative careers. In C. B. Fisher & R. M. Lerner (Eds.), *Applied developmental psychology* (pp. 502-522). New York: McGraw-Hill.
Lerner, R. M., & Kauffman, M. B. (1985). The concept of development in contextualism. *Developmental Review, 5,* 309-333.
Lerner, R. M., & Knapp, J.R. (1975). Actual and perceived intrafamilial attitudes of late adolescents and their parents. *Journal of Youth and Adolescence, 4,* 17-36.
Lerner, R. M., & Lerner, J.V. (1989). Organismic and social contextual bases of development: The sample case of early adolescence. In W. Damon (Ed.), *Child development today and tomorrow* (pp. 69-85). San Francisco: Jossey-Bass.
Lerner, R. M., & Miller, J. R. (1993). Integrating human development research and intervention for America's children: The Michigan State University model. *Journal of Applied Developmental Psychology, 14,* 347-364.
Lerner, R. M., Miller, J. R., Knott, J. H., Corey, K. E., Bynum, T. S., Hoopfer, L. C., McKinney, M. H., Abrams, L. A., Hula, R. C., & Terry, P. A. (1994). Integrating scholarship and outreach in human development research, policy, and service: A developmental contextual perspective. In D. L. Featherman, R. M. Lerner, & M. Perlmutter (Eds.), *Life-span development and behavior, 12* (pp. 249-273). Hillsdale, NJ: Erlbaum.
Lerner, R. M., Miller, J. R., & Ostrom, C. W. (1995, Spring). Integrative knowledge, accountability, access, and the American university of the twenty-first century: A family and consumer sciences vision of the future of higher education. *Kappa Omicron Nu FORUM, 8*(1), 11-27.
Lerner, R. M., Petersen, A. C., & Brooks-Gunn, J. (Eds.). (1991). *Encyclopedia of adolescence.* New York: Garland.

Lerner, R. M., Ostrom, C. W., & Freel, M. A. (1995). Promoting positive youth and community development through outreach scholarship: Comments on Zeldin and Peterson. *Journal of Adolescent Research, 10*, 486-502.

Lerner, R. M., & Ryff, C. D. (1978). Implementation of the life-span view of human development: The sample case of attachment. In P. B. Baltes (Ed.), *Life-span development and behavior* (Vol. 12, pp. 1-44). New York: Academic Press.

Lerner, R. M., & Simon, L. A. K. (1998a). The new American outreach university: Challenges and options. In R. M. Lerner & L. A. K. Simon (Eds.), *University-community collaborations for the twenty-first century: Outreach scholarship for youth and familes* (pp. 3-23). New York: Garland.

Lerner, R. M., & Simon, L. A. K. (Eds.). (1998b). *University-community collaborations for the twenty-first century: Outreach scholarship for youth and families.* New York: Garland.

Lerner, R. M., & Spanier, G. B. (Eds.) (1978). *Child influences on marital and family interaction: A life span perspective.* New York: Academic Press.

Lerner, R. M., & Spanier, G. B. (1980). *Adolescent development: A life-span perspective.* New York: McGraw-Hill.

Lerner, R. M., & Tubman, J. (1989). Conceptual issues in studying continuity and discontinuity in personality development across life. *Journal of Personality, 57*, 343-373.

Lewin, K. (1943). Psychology and the process of group living. *Journal of Social Psychology, 17*, 113-131.

Lewis, M. (1997). *Altering fate.* New York: Guilford Press.

Lewontin, R. C. (1981). On constraints and adaptation. *Behavioral and Brain Science, 4*, 244-245.

Lewontin, R. C., Rose, S., & Kamin, L. J. (1984). *Not in our genes: Biology, ideology, and human nature.* New York: Pantheon Press.

Little, R. R. (1993, March). *What's working for today's youth: The issues, the programs, and the learnings.* Paper presented at an ICYF Fellows Colloquium, Michigan State University, East Lansing.

Lord, S. E., Eccles, J. S., & McCarthy, K. A. (1994). Surviving the junior high school transition: Family processes and self-perceptions as protective and risk factors. *Journal of Early Adolescence, 14*, 162-199.

Lorenz, K. (1965). *Evolution and modification of behavior.* Chicago: University of Chicago Press.

Luster, T., & McAdoo, H. P. (1994). Factors related to the achievement and adjustment of young African American children. *Child Development, 65*, 1080-1094.

Luster, T., & McAdoo, H. (1996). Family and child influences on educational attainment: A secondary analysis of the High/Scope Perry Preschool data. *Developmental Psychology, 32*(1), 26-39.

Maccoby, E., & Martin, J. (1983). Socialization in the context of the family: Parent-child interaction. In E. M. Hetherington (Ed.), *Handbook of child psychology: Socialization, personality, and social development* (Vol. 4, pp. 1-101). New York: Wiley.

Maggs, J. L., & Galambos, N.L. (1993). Alternative structural models for understanding adolescent problem behavior in two-earner families. *Journal of Early Adolescence, 13*(1), 79-101.

Mason, C. A., Cauce, A. M., Gonzales, N., & Hiraga, Y. (1994). Adolescent problem behavior: The effects of peers on the moderating role of father absence and the mother-child relationship. *American Journal of Community Psychology, 22*, 723-743.

Masters, R. D. (1978). Jean-Jacques is alive and well: Rousseau and contemporary sociobiology. *Daedalus, 107*, 93-105.

Matute-Bianchi, M. E. (1986). Ethnic identities and patterns of school success and failures among Mexican-descent and Japanese American students in a California high school: An ethnographic analysis. Special Issue: The education of Hispanic Americans: A challenge for the future. *American Journal of Education, 95*, 233-255.

McAdoo, H. P. (1977). A review of the literature related to family therapy in the Black community. *Journal of Contemporary Psychotherapy, 9*, 15-19.

McAdoo, H. P. (1981). Upward mobility and parenting in middle-income Black families. *The Journal of Black Psychology, 8*, 1-22.

McAdoo, H. P. (1982). Stress absorbing systems in Black families. *Family Relations, 31*, 479-488.

McAdoo, H. (1991). Family values and outcomes for children. *Journal of Negro Education, 60*, 361-365.

McAdoo, H. (1992). Reaffirming African-American families and our identities. *Psychology Discourse, 23*(3), 6-7.

McAdoo, H.P. (1993). *Family ethnicity: Strength in diversity.* Newbury Park, CA: Sage.

McAdoo, H. (1998a). African American families: Strength and realities. In H. McCubbin, E. Thompson, & J. Futrell, (Eds.), *Resiliency in ethnic minority families: African American families* (pp. 17-30). Thousand Oaks, CA: Sage.

McAdoo, H. P. (1998b). African-American families. In C. H. Mindel, R. W. Habenstein, & W. Roosevelt, Jr., (Eds.), *Ethnic families in America: Patterns and variations* (4th ed., pp. 361-381). Upper Saddle River, NJ: Prentice Hall.

McAdoo, H. P. (1999). Diverse children of color. In H. E. Fitzgerald, B. M. Lester, & B. S. Zuckerman (Eds.), *Children of color: Research, health, and policy issues* (pp. 205-218). New York: Garland Publishing.

McAdoo, H. P., & Crawford, V. (1991). *The Black Church and family support programs. Families as nurturing systems: Support across the life span* (pp. 193-222). New York: Haworth Press.
McCubbin, H. I., Fleming, W. M., Thompson, A. I., Neitman, P., Elver, K., & Savas, S.A. (1998). Resiliency and coping in "at risk" African-American youth and their families. In H. I. McCubbin, E. A. Thompson, A. I. Thompson, & J. E. Futrell (Eds.), *Resiliency in ethnic minority families: African-American families* (Vol.2, pp. 287-328). Thousand Oaks, CA: Sage.
McCubbin, H. I., Futrell, J. A., Thompson, E.A., & Thompson, A. I. (1998). Resilient families in an ethnic and cultural context. In H. I. McCubbin, E. A. Thompson, A. I. Thompson, & J. E. Futrell (Eds.), *Resiliency in ethnic minority families: African-American families* (Vol.2, pp. 329-351). Thousand Oaks, CA: Sage.
McKnight, J. L., & Kretzmann, J. P. (1993). Mapping community capacity. *Michigan State University Community and Economic Development Program Community News* (pp. 1-4).
McLanahan, S., & Booth, K. (1989). Mother-only families: Problems, prospects, and policies. *Journal of Marriage and the Family, 51*, 557-580.
McLanahan, S., & Sandefur, G. D. (1994). *Uncertain childhood, uncertain future.* Cambridge, MA: Harvard University Press.
McLoyd, V. C. (1990). Minority children: Introduction to the Special Issue. *Child Development, 61*, 263-266.
McLoyd, V. C. (1994). Research in the service of poor and ethnic/racial minority children: A moral imperative. *Family and Consumer Sciences Research Journal, 23*, 56-66.
McLoyd, V. C., & Wilson, L. (1991). The strain of living poor: Parenting, social support, and child mental health. In A. C. Huston (Ed.), *Children in poverty: Child development and public policy* (pp. 105-135). Cambridge: Cambridge University Press.
Melby, J. N., & Conger, R. D. (1996). Parental behaviors and adolescent academic performance: A longitudinal analysis. *Journal of Research on Adolescence, 6*(1), 113-137.
Meyers, M. K. (1993). Child care in JOBS employment and training program: What difference does quality make? *Journal of Marriage and the Family, 55*, 767-783.
Miller, J. R., & Lerner, R. M. (1994). Integrating research and outreach: Developmental contextualism and the human ecological perspective. *Home Economics Forum, 7*, 21-28.
Mindel, C. H., Habenstein, R. W., & Roosevelt, W., Jr. (Eds.). (1998). *Ethnic families in America: Patterns and variations* (4th ed.). Upper Saddle River, NJ: Prentice Hall.
Moffitt, R. (1992). Incentive effects in the U.S. welfare system: A review. *Journal of Economic Literature, 30*, 1-61.
Moore, K. A. (1992, June). *Our nation's children.* Testimony presented before the U.S. House of Representatives Subcommittee on Census and Population Committee on Post Office and Civil Service. (Available from Child Trends, Inc., 2100 M Street NW, Suite 610, Washington, DC 20037.)
Moore, K. A. (1994, June 23). *Teenage childbearing and welfare.* Washington, D.C.: Child Trends.
Moore, K., Morrison, D. R., Zaslow, M., & Glei, D. A. (1994). *Ebbing and flowing, learning and growing: Family economic resources and children's development.* Paper presented at research briefing, Board on Children and Families, December 5-6, 1994. Washington, D.C.: Child Trends, Inc.
Moore, K. A., & Snyder, N. O. (1994). *Facts at a glance.* Washington, D.C.: Child Trends.
Morelli, G. A., & Verhoef, H. (in press). Who should help me raise my child. In C. Le Monda & L. Balter (Eds.), *Handbook of child psychology.* New York: Garland.
Muller, C. (1995). Maternal employment, parent involvement, and mathematics achievement among adolescents. *Journal of Marriage and the Family, 57*, 85-100.
Murray, C. (1984). *Losing ground: American social policy, 1950-1980.* New York: Basic Books.
National Center for Children in Poverty. (1998). Young children poverty in the States--Wide variation and significant change. *Childhood Poverty (Research Brief 1).* New York: Columbia University School of Public Health.
National Commission on America's Urban Families. (1993). *Families first.* Washington, DC: Author.
National Research Council. (1993). *Losing generations: Adolescents in high-risk settings.* Washington, DC: National Academy Press.
Nightingale, D. S., & Holcomb, P. A. (1997). Alternative strategies for increasing employment. In K. Bogenschneider, T. Corbett, M. E. Bell, & K. D. Linney, (Eds.), *Moving families out of poverty: Employment, tax, and investment strategies. Wisconsin Family Impact Seminars and the Institute for Research on Poverty Briefing Report* (pp. 1-14). Madison, WI: School of Human Ecology, University of Wisconsin-Madison.
Nisbet, R. A. (1980). *History of the idea of progress.* New York: Basic Books.
Novikoff, A. B. (1945). The concept of integrative levels of biology. *Science, 62*, 209-215.
Office of Hawaiian Affairs. (1994). *Native Hawaiian data book.* Honolulu: Office of Hawaiian Affairs.
Office of Special Education, Department of Education. (1995). *16th annual report to Congress: Study of special populations of Native American students with disabilities*, 195-230.
O'Leary, W. (1998, November 23). *Coordination of health and human services agencies.* Presentation to Family and Health Care Working Group of Governor Cellucci's Transition Team. Boston Medical Center, Boston, MA.

Ooms, T. (1992). *Families in poverty: Patterns, contexts, and implications for policy.* Washington, D.C.: The Family Impact Seminar.

Ostrom, C. W., Lerner, R. M., & Freel, M. A. (1995). Building the capacity of youth and families through university-community collaborations: The development-in-context evaluation (DICE) model. *Journal of Adolescent Research, 10,* 427-448.

Overton, W. F. (1998). Developmental psychology: Philosophy, concepts, and methodology. In W. Damon (Series Ed.) & R. M. Lerner (Vol. Ed.), *Handbook of child psychology: Vol. 1 Theoretical models of human development* (5th ed., pp. 107-187). New York: Wiley.

Papini, D. R., & Roggman, L. A. (1992). Adolescent perceived attachment to parents in relation to competence, depression, and anxiety: A longitudinal study. *Journal of Early Adolescence, 12*(4), 420-440.

Papini, D. R., Roggman, L. A., & Anderson, J. (1991). Early-adolescent perceptions of attachment to mother and father: A test of the emotional-distancing and buffering hypotheses. *Journal of Early Adolescence, 11*(2), 258-275.

Paulson, S. E. (1994). Relations of parenting style and parental involvement with ninth-grade students' achievement. *Journal of Early Adolescence, 14,* 250-267.

Paulson, S. E., Hill, J. P., & Holmbeck, G. N. (1991). Distinguishing between perceived closeness and parental warmth in families with seventh-grade boys and girls. *Journal of Early Adolescence, 11,* 276-293.

Peterson, P. L., Hawkins, J. D., Abbott, R. D., & Catalano, R. F. (1994). Disentangling the effects of parental drinking, family management, and parental alcohol norms on current drinking by black and white adolescents. *Journal of Research on Adolescence, 4*(2), 203-277.

Phillips, D. A. (Ed.). (1995). *Child care for low-income families: Summary of two workshops.* Washington, D.C.: National Academy Press.

Phillips, D. A., & Bridgman, A. (Eds.). (1995). *New findings on children, families, and economic self-sufficiency: summary of a research briefing.* Washington, D.C.: National Academy Press.

Phillips, D., & Bridgman, A. (Eds.). (1997). *New findings on welfare and children's development: Summary of a research briefing.* Washington DC: National Academy Press.

Phinney, J. S., & Chavira, V. (1992). Ethnic identity and self-esteem: An exploratory longitudinal study. *Journal of Adolescence, 15,* 271-281.

Phinney, J. S., & Chavira, V. (1995). Parental ethnic socialization and adolescent coping with problems related to ethnicity. *Journal of Research on Adolescence, 5*(1), 31-54.

Piaget, J. (1950). *The psychology of intelligence.* New York: Harcourt Brace.

Piaget, J. (1970). Piaget's theory. In P. H. Mussen (Ed.), *Carmichael's manual of child psychology* (3rd ed., Vol. 1, pp. 703-723). New York: Wiley.

Piaget, J. (1972). Intellectual evolution from adolescence to adulthood. *Human Development, 15,* 1-12.

Pike, A., McGuire, S., Hetherington, E. M., Reiss, D., & Plomin, R. (1996). Family environment and adolescent depressive symptoms and antisocial behavior: A multivariate genetic analysis. *Developmental Psychology, 32*(4), 574-589.

Pittman, K. J., & Irby, M. (1996). *Promoting life skills for youth: Beyond indicators for survival and problem prevention.* Baltimore, MD: International Youth Foundation.

Pittman, K. J., & Zeldin, S. (1994). From deterrence to development: Shifting the focus of youth programs for African-American males. In R. B. Mincy (Ed.), *Nurturing young black males: Challenges to agencies, programs, and social policy* (pp. 45-55). Washington, DC: The Urban Institute Press.

Plomin, R. (1986). *Development, genetics, and psychology.* Hillsdale, NJ: Erlbaum.

Reddy, M. (1993). *Statistical records of Native North Americans.* Detroit: Gale Research.

Renick, M. J., Blumberg, S. L., & Markman, H. J. (1992). The prevention and relationship enhancement program (PREP): An empirically based prevention intervention program for couples. *Family Relations, 41,* 141-147.

Richards, M.H., & Duckett, E. (1994). The relationship of maternal employment to early adolescent daily experience with and without parents. *Child Development, 65,* 225-236.

Riegel, K. F. (1975). Toward a dialectical theory of development. *Human Development, 18,* 50-64.

Riegel, K. F. (1976a). The dialectics of human development. *American Psychologist, 31,* 689-700.

Riegel, K. F. (1976b). From traits and equilibrium toward developmental dialectics. In W. J. Arnold & J. K. Cole (Eds.), *Nebraska symposium on motivation* (pp. 348-408). Lincoln: University of Nebraska.

Robinson, W., Ruch-Ross, H. S., Watkins-Ferrell, P., & Lightfoot, S. L. (1993). Risk behavior in adolescents: Methodological challenges in school-based research. *School Psychology Quarterly, 8,* 241-254.

Roth, J., Brooks-Gunn, J., Galen, B., Murray, L., Silverman, P., Liu, H., Man, D., & Foster, W. (1997). *Promoting healthy adolescence: Youth development frameworks and programs.* New York: Teachers College, Columbia University.

Rowe, D. C. (1994). *The limits of family influence: Genes, experience, and behavior.* New York: Guilford Press.

Rubenstein, J. L., & Feldman, S. S. (1993). Conflict-resolution behavior in adolescent boys: Antecedents and adaptational correlates. *Journal of Research on Adolescence, 3*(1), 41-66.

Rueter, M. A., & Conger, R. D. (1995). Interaction style, problem-solving behavior, and family problem-solving effectiveness. *Child Development, 66*, 98-115.
Sahlins, M. D. (1976). *The use and abuse of biology.* Ann Arbor, MI: The University of Michigan Press.
Sam, D. L. (1995). Acculturation attitudes among young immigrants as a function of perceived parental attitudes toward cultural change. *Journal of Early Adolescence, 15*(2), 238-258.
Sameroff, A. J. (1983). Developmental systems: Contexts and evolution. In W. Kessen (Ed.), *Handbook of child psychology: Vol. 1, History, theory, and methods* (pp. 237-294). New York: Wiley.
Sameroff, A. J., Seifer, R., Baldwin, A., & Baldwin, C. (1993). Stability of intelligence from preschool to adolescence: The influence of social and family risk factors. *Child Development, 64*, 80-97.
Scales, P., & Leffert, N. (1999). *Developmental assets: A synthesis of the scientific research on adolescent development.* Minneapolis, MN: Search Institute.
Schaie, K. W. (1979). The primary mental abilities in adulthood: An exploration in the development of psychometric intelligence. In P. B. Baltes & O. G. Brim Jr. (Eds.), *Life-span development and behavior, 2* (pp. 67-115). New York: Academic.
Schneirla, T. C. (1957). The concept of development in comparative psychology. In D. B. Harris (Ed.), *The concept of development* (pp. 78-108). Minneapolis, MN: University of Minnesota.
Schorr, L. B. (1988). *Within our reach: Breaking the cycle of disadvantage.* New York: Doubleday.
Schorr, L. (1997). *Common purpose: Strengthening families and neighborhoods to rebuild America.* New York: Doubleday.
Scott-Jones, D., & White, A. B. (1990). Correlates of sexual activity in early adolescence. *Journal of Early Adolescence, 10*(2), 221-238.
Seltzer, J. (1994). *Child support and fairness.* Presentation at the annual meeting of the National Council on Family Relations, Minneapolis, MN.
Shagle, S. C., & Barber, B. K. (1993). Effects of family, marital, and parent-child conflict on adolescent self-derogation and suicidal ideation. *Journal of Marriage and the Family, 55*, 964-974.
Simmons, R. G., & Blyth, D. A. (1987). *Moving into adolescence: The impact of pubertal change and school context.* Hawthorne, NJ: Aldine.
Simons, J. M., Finlay, B., & Yang, A. (1991). *The adolescent and young adult fact book.* Washington, DC: Children's Defense Fund.
Simons, R. L., Johnson, C., & Conger, R. D. (1994). Harsh corporal punishment versus quality of parental involvement as an explanation of adolescent maladjustment. *Journal of Marriage and the Family, 56*, 591-607.
Small, S. A., & Kerns, D. (1993). Unwanted sexual activity among peers during early and middle adolescence: Incidence and risk factors. *Journal of Marriage and the Family, 55*, 941-952.
Small, S. A., & Luster, T. (1994). An ecological risk-factor approach to adolescent sexual activity. *Journal of Marriage and the Family, 56*, 181-192.
Smetana, J. G. (1993). Conceptions of parental authority in divorced and married mothers and their adolescents. *Journal of Research on Adolescence, 3*(1), 19-39.
Smetana, J. G., Yau, J. & Hanson, S. (1991). Conflict resolution in families with adolescents. *Journal of Research on Adolescence, 1*(2), 189-206.
Smith, S. (Ed.). (1995). *Two generation programs for families in poverty: A new intervention strategy.* Norwood, NJ: Ablex.
Smith, S. (Ed.). (1997). *The well-being of children in working poor families.* New York: Foundation for Child Development.
Smith, S., Blank, S., & Collins, R. (1992). *Pathways to self-sufficiency for two generations: Designing welfare-to-work programs that benefit children and strengthen families.* New York: Foundation for Child Development.
Smith, S. L., Fairchild, M., & Groginsky, S. (1997). *Early childhood care and education.* Denver: National Conference of State Legislatures.
Smith, S., & Zaslow, M. (1995). Rationale and policy context for two-generation intervention. In S. Smith (Ed.), *Two-generation programs for families in poverty.* Norwood, NJ: Ablex.
Sparks, E. (1996). The challenges facing community health centers in the 1990s: A voice from the inner city. In M. B. Lykes, A. Banuazizi, R. Liem, & M. Morris (Eds.), *Myths about the powerless: Contesting social inequalities* (pp. 237-257). Philadelphia: Temple University Press.
Spencer, M. B. (1983). Children's cultural values and parental child-rearing strategies. *Developmental Review, 3*, 51-370.
Spencer, M. B. (1984). Black children's race awareness, racial attitudes, and self-concept: A reinterpretation. *Journal of Child Psychology & Psychiatry & Allied Disciplines, 25*, 433-441.
Spencer, M. B. (1987). Black children's ethnic identity formation: Risk and resilience of castelike minorities. In J. S. Phinney & M. J. Rotheram (Eds.), *Children's ethnic socialization: Pluralism and development* (pp. 103-116). Newbury Park, CA: Sage Publications.
Spencer, M. B. (1990). Development of minority children: An introduction. *Child Development, 61*, 267-269.
Steinberg, L. (1987). The impact of puberty on family relations: Effects of pubertal status and pubertal timing. *Developmental Psychology, 23*, 833-840.

Steinberg, L., Mounts, N. S., Lamborn, S. D., & Dornbusch, S. M. (1991). Authoritative parenting and adolescent adjustment across varied ecological niches. *Journal of Research on Adolescence, 1*(1), 19-36.

Stice, E., & Barrera, J. (1995). A longitudinal examination of the reciprocal relations between perceived parenting and adolescents' substance use and externalizing behaviors. *Developmental Psychology, 31*(2), 322-334.

Sullivan, M. L. (1993). Culture and class as determinants of out-of-wedlock childbearing and poverty during late adolescence. *Journal of Research on Adolescence, 3*(3), 295-316.

Taylor, R. D. (1996). Adolescents' perceptions of kinship support and family management practices: Association with adolescent adjustment in African American families. *Developmental Psychology, 32*(4), 687-695.

Taylor, R., & Roberts, D. (1995). Kinship support and maternal and adolescent well-being in economically disadvantaged African-American families. *Child Development, 66*, 1585-1597.

Taylor Gibbs, J., & Huang, L. N. (1998). *Children of color: Psychological interventions with culturally diverse youth.* San Francisco, CA: Jossey-Bass Publishers.

Thelen, E., & Smith, L. B. (1994). *A dynamic systems approach to the development of cognition and action.* Cambridge, MA: MIT Press.

Thelen, E., & Smith, L. B. (1998). Dynamic systems theories. In W. Damon (Series Ed.) and R. M. Lerner (Vol. Ed.), *Handbook of child psychology: Vol. 1 Theoretical models of human development* (5th ed., pp. 563-633). New York: Wiley.

Thomas, A., & Chess, S. (1977). *Temperament and development.* New York: Brunner/Mazel.

Tobach, E. (1981). Evolutionary aspects of the activity of the organism and its development. In R. M. Lerner & N. A. Busch-Rossnagel (Eds.), *Individuals as producers of their development: A lifespan perspective* (pp. 37-68). New York: Academic.

Tobach, E., & Greenberg, G. (1984). The significance of T. C. Schneirla's contribution to the concept of levels of integration. In G. Greenberg & E. Tobach (Eds.), *Behavioral evolution and integrative levels* (pp. 1-7). Hillsdale, NJ: Erlbaum.

Tobach, E., & Schneirla, T. C. (1968). The biopsychology of social behavior of animals. In R. E. Cooke & S. Levin (Eds.), *Biologic basis of pediatric practice* (pp. 68-82). New York: McGraw-Hill.

Tubman, J. G., & Lerner, R. M. (1994). Affective experiences of parents and their children from adolescence to young adulthood: Stability of affective experiences. *Journal of Adolescence, 17*, 81-98.

Turner, R. A., Irwin, C. E., & Millstein, S. G. (1991). Family structure, family processes, and experimenting with substances during adolescence. *Journal of Research on Adolescence, 1*(1), 93-106.

United States Department of Commerce. (1991, August). *Poverty in the United States: 1990* (Current Population Reports, Series P-60, No. 175). Washington, DC: U.S. Government Printing Office.

United States Department of Commerce. (1993). *Poverty in the United States: 1993* (Current Population Reports, Series P-60, No. 178). Washington, DC: U.S. Government Printing Office.

United States Department of Health and Human Services. (1996). *Trends in the well-being of America's children and youth: 1996.* Washington, DC: Department on Health and Human Services, Office of the Secretary for Planning and Evaluation.

Ventura, S. J., Martin, J. A., & Taffel, S. M. (1994). Advance report of final natality statistics, 1992. *Monthly Vital Statistics Report, 43* (5, suppl.). Hyattsville, MD: National Center for Health Statistics.

Vinovskis, M. A. (1988). *An "epidemic" of adolescent pregnancy?: Some historical and policy considerations.* New York: Oxford University Press.

Wallerstein, J.S. (1986). Children of divorce: Preliminary report of a ten-year follow-up of older children and adolescents. In S. Chess & A. Thomas (Eds.), *Annual progress in child psychiatry and child development.* New York: Brunner/Mazel, Inc.

Wallerstein, J. S., & Blakeslee, S. (1989). *Second chances: Men, women, and children a decade after divorce.* New York: Ticknor & Fields.

Walsten, D. (1990). Insensitivity of the analysis of variance to heredity-environment interaction. *Behavioral and Brain Sciences, 13*, 109-120.

Wapner, S. (1993). Parental development: A holistic, developmental systems-oriented perspective. In J. Demick, K. Bursik, & R. DiBiase (Eds.), *Parental development* (pp. 3-37). Hillsdale, NJ: Erlbaum.

Wapner, S., & Demick, J. (1998). Developmental analysis: A holistic, developmental, systems-oriented perspective. In W. Damon (Series Ed.) and R. M. Lerner (Vol. Ed.), *Handbook of child psychology: Vol. 1 Theoretical models of human development* (5th ed., pp. 761-805). New York: Wiley.

Washburn, S. L. (Ed.). (1961). *Social life of early men.* New York: Wenner-Gren Foundation for Anthropological Research.

Weiss, H. B., & Greene, J. C. (1992). An empowerment partnership for family support and education programs and evaluations. *Family Science Review, 5*, 131-148.

Weller, A., Florian, V., & Mikulincer, M. (1995). Adolescents' reports on parental division of power in a multicultural society. *Journal of Research on Adolescence, 5*(4), 413-429.

Wentzel, K. R., Feldman, S. S., & Weinberger, D. A. (1991). Parental child rearing and academic achievement in boys: The mediational role of social-emotional adjustment. *Journal of Early Adolescence, 11*(3), 321-339.

Werner, E. E., & Smith, R. S. (1982). *Vulnerable but invincible: A longitudinal study of resilient children and youth.* New York: McGraw-Hill.

Werner, E. E., & Smith, R. S. (1992). *Overcoming the odds: High risk children from birth to adulthood.* Ithaca, NY: Cornell University Press.

Werner, H. (1957). The concept of development from a comparative and organismic point of view. In D. B. Harris (Ed.), *The concept of development* (pp. 125-148). Minneapolis: University of Minnesota.

Wetzel, J. (1987). *American youth: A statistical snapshot.* New York: William T. Grant Foundation.

Whitbeck, L. B. (1987). Modeling efficacy: The effect of perceived parental efficacy on the self-efficacy of early adolescents. *Journal of Early Adolescence, 7*(2), 165-177.

Whitbeck, L. B., Simons, R. L., & Kao, M. (1994). The effects of divorced mothers' dating behaviors and sexual attitudes on the sexual attitudes and behaviors of their adolescent children. *Journal of Marriage and the Family, 56,* 615-621.

Wilcox, B. (1994). *Welfare incentives and teen childbearing: Do the facts fit the political fury?* Center on Children, Families and the Law, University of Nebraska, 121 South 13th, Suite 302, Lincoln, NE 68588-0227.

Wilson, M. N. (Ed.). (1995). African American family life: Its structural and ecological aspects. *New Directions for Child Development, 68.*

Wilson, M. N., Phillip, D. G., Kohn, L. P., & Curry-El, J. A. (1995). Cultural relativistic approach toward ethnic minorities in family therapy. In J. Aponte, R. Young Rivers, & J. Wohl (Eds.), *Psychological interventions and cultural diversity* (pp. 92-108). Boston: Allyn & Bacon.

Wright, D. W., Peterson, L., & Barnes, H. L. (1990). The relation of parental employment and contextual variables with sexual permissiveness and gender role attitudes of rural early adolescents. *Journal of Early Adolescence, 10*(3), 382-398.

Wulczyn, F. (1994). Status at birth and infant foster care placement in New York City. In R. Barth, J. D. Berrick, & N. Gilbert (Eds.), *Child welfare research review, Vol. 1* (pp. 146-184). New York: Columbia University Press.

Yax, L. K. (1998). *National estimates: Annual population estimates by age group and sex, selected years from 1990 to 1998.* Washington, D.C.: U.S. Census Bureau.

Young, M. H., Miller, B. C., Norton, M. C., & Hill, E. J. (1995). The effect of parental supportive behaviors on life satisfaction of adolescent offspring. *Journal of Marriage and the Family, 57,* 813-822.

Zabin, L. S., Astone, N. M., & Emerson, M. R. (1993). Do adolescents want babies? The relationship between attitudes and behavior. *Journal of Research on Adolescence, 3,* 67-86.

Zaslow, M. J. (1988). Sex differences in children's response to parental divorce: I. Research methodology and postdivorce family forms. *American Journal of Orthopsychiatry, 58*(3), 355-378.

Zaslow, M. J. (1989). Sex differences in children's response to parental divorce: II. Samples, variables, ages, and sources. *American Journal of Orthopsychiatry, 59*(1), 118-141.

Zaslow, M. J., & Eldred, C. A. (Eds.). (1998). *Parenting behavior in a sample of young mothers in poverty: Results of the New Chance Observational Study.* New York: Manpower Demonstration Research Corporation.

Zaslow, M., Tout, K., Smith, S., & Moore, K. (1998). Implications of the 1996 welfare legislation for children: A research perspective. *Social Policy Report, Society for Research in Child Development, 12*(3).

Zeldin, S. (1995). *Opportunities and supports for youth development: Lessons from research implications for community leaders and scholars.* Washington, D.C.: Center for Youth Development and Policy Research, Academy for Educational Development.

Zigler, E., & Finn-Stevenson, M. (1992). Applied developmental psychology. In M. H. Bornstein & M. E. Lamb (Eds.), *Developmental psychology: An advanced textbook* (3rd ed., pp. 677-729). Hillsdale, NJ: Erlbaum.

Zill, N. (1983, March). *Divorce, marital conflict, and children's mental health: Research findings and policy recommendations.* Testimony presented before the U.S. Senate Subcommittee on Family and Human Services. (Available from Child Trends, Inc., 2100 M Street NW, Suite 610, Washington, DC 20037.)

Zill, N., Moore, K. A., Smith, E. W., Stief, T., & Coiro, M. J. (1991). *The life circumstances and development of children in welfare families: A profile based on national survey data.* Washington, D. C.: Child Trends.

Zill, N, Morrison, D.R., & Coiro, M.J. (1993). Long-term effects of parental divorce on parent child relationships, adjustment, and achievement in young adulthood. *Journal of Family Psychology, 7,* 91-103.

Zimiles, H., & Lee, V. (1991). Adolescent family structure and educational progress. *Developmental Psychology, 27*(2), 314-320.

Zimmerman, M. A., Ramirez, J. Washienko, K. M., Walter, B, & Dyer, S. (1998). Enculturation hypothesis: Exploring direct and protective effects among Native American youth. In H. I. McCubbin, E. A. Thompson, A. I. Thompson, & J. E. Fromer (Eds.), *Resiliency in ethnic minority families: Native and immigrant American families* (Vol. 1, pp. 199-220). Thousand Oaks, CA: Sage.

Zimmerman, M., Salem, D., & Maton, K. (1995). Family structure and psychosocial correlates among urban African-American adolescent males. *Child Development, 66*, 1598-1613.

Name Index

Abbott, R. D., 69
Aber, M. S., 22
Abramovitz, M., 104
Abrams, L. A., 32,39,127,131
Acock, A. A., 69
Adelson, J., 65
Ahlburg, D. A., 3
Almeida, D. M., 64,67,71
Anderson, J., 67
Andrews, J. A., 69
Allison, K. W., 3-4, 19-20, 91
Antonucci, T. C., 125-129
Arbreton, A. J., 65
Armistead, L., 70
Arthur, J., 129
Ary, D. V., 69
Astone, N. M., 75
Axinn, J. M., 86

Baer, D. M., 23-34, 37
Baldwin, A., 69
Baldwin, C., 69
Baltes, P. B., 25, 30, 33, 35-37, 39, 129
Bare, M. J., 85, 97-100
Barber, B. K., 67-68
Bannes, H. L., 70
Barnes, G. M., 67
Barrera, J., 69
Barrera, M., 69
Barringer, F., 43
Baumrind, D., 63-64, 68
Bell, M.E., 58, 80
Belsky, J., 63
Bennett, H., 15
Benson, P. L., 59, 66, 102, 111, 113-117, 120-121, 126, 140
Best, K. M., 66, 68-69

Bijou, S. W., 32-35, 37
Bingham, C. R., 75
Birkel, R., 34,39
Blakeslee, S., 102
Blank, H., 92
Blank, S., 58, 80-81, 89-90
Blum, B. B., 58, 86, 89
Blumberg, S. L., 103
Blyth, D. A., 111, 113-117, 129
Bogenschneider, K., 58, 79-81, 84, 87, 89, 94, 106-107
Booth, K., 101-102
Bornstein, M. H., 62
Bowlby, J., 32
Bowman, H. A., 109
Boyer, E. L., 134
Brabeck, M. M., 67
Brandtstädter, J., 38
Brennan, M., 40
Bridgman, A., 13, 88, 91-93
Brim, O. G., 27, 35-36
Briones, M., 66
Brodkin, K., 51
Bronfenbrenner, U., 25, 27, 29, 34, 36-38, 40-41, 44, 132-133, 138
Brooks-Gunn, J., 38, 119-126
Bronstein, P., 66
Brown, B. B., 64
Brown, N. L., 75
Buchanan, C. M., 70
Bumpass, L., 11
Burkam, D. T., 70
Burton, L. M., 48,90-91
Bush, N. F., 69
Busch-Rossnagel, N. A., 36-37
Bynum, T. S., 32, 39, 127, 131

Cairns, R. C., 32, 35, 41, 136

Canning, R. D., 75
Carson, A., 69
Castellino, D. R., 3, 4, 37, 49, 58, 61-62, 81, 91
Catalano, R. F., 69
Cauce, A. M., 22, 68
Ceci, S. J., 37-38, 40, 133
Chansky, T. E., 38
Chassin, L., 69
Chavira, V., 45, 65
Chen, C., 69
Cherlin, A. J., 70, 103
Chess, S., 28, 36, 129
Chibucos, T., 139
Chiu, M. L., 65
Coiro, M. J., 81, 101
Collins, R., 58, 80-81, 89-90.
Compass, B. F., 68
Conger, R. D., 64, 66, 68-69
Corbett, T., 5-8, 79-80, 82, 85-87, 90, 93-99, 103, 105-107, 110
Corkey, K. E., 32, 39, 127, 131.
Costa, F. M., 75
Cox, M., 69-70
Cox, R., 69-70
Crawford, V., 56-57
Crnic, K., 30-31
Crockett, L., 75
Crouter, A. C., 25
Crystal, D. S. 64
Csikszentmihalyi, M., 38
Curry, J. A., 47

Damon, W., 59, 140
D'Angelo, L. L., 68
Darling, N., 64
Darwin, C., 35
Davidson, C. E., 96
Davies, M. W., 88-89, 93
Denzik, J., 23
Demo, D. H., 69
De Vita, C. J., 3
di Mauro, D., 72
Dixon, R. A., 32
Doherty, W. J., 69-70
Donovan, J. E., 75

Dornbusch, S. M., 63, 65, 70
Drake, D. R., 111, 113-116
Dryfoos, J. B., 18, 43, 58, 77, 109, 119, 124, 127, 137
Dubois, D.V., 67
Duckett, E., 71
Duncan, G. J., 105
Durbin, D. V., 64
Duvall, E. M., 129
Dyer, S., 45

East, P. L., 67, 75
Eccles, J. S., 65-66, 71
Eddey, M. A., 109
Eisenberg, N., 66
Eitel, S. K., 67
Elder, G. H., 25-26, 30, 35, 44, 140
Eldred, C. A., 88-89
Ellwood, J. T., 85, 97-100
Elver, K., 22
Emerson, M. R., 75
Emler, N. P., 28
Erickson, J. B., 34-35, 122
Erikson, E. H., 32, 129

Fairchild, M., 19, 58, 80
Farrell, M. P., 67
Featherman, D. L., 4, 28
Feldman, S. S., 64-65, 68, 75
Felice, M. E., 75
Felner, R. D., 22, 67
Fine, M. A., 70
Finley, B., 16, 17, 66, 68
Finn-Stevenson, M., 44, 136
Finkelstein, J. W., 28-29
Fisher, C. B., 34, 38, 40-41, 53, 67, 127, 134
Fitzgerald, M., 66
Fitzsimmons, E., 84, 87, 106
Flanagan, C. A., 71
Fleming, W. M., 22
Flor, D., 67
Florian, V., 65
Ford, D. H., 25, 29, 33-34, 37, 61, 127
Forehand, R., 69-70
Fortenberry, J. D., 75

Family Diversity and Family Policy

Foster, W., 119-126
Freedman-Doan, C. R., 65
Freedman, D. G., 34
Freel, M. A., 130, 136
Freud, A., 32, 129
Freud, S., 32-33, 37
Furstenberg, F. F., 70, 103

Galambos, N. L., 64, 67-68, 70-71
Galen, B., 119-126
García Coll, C., 30-31
Garfinkel, I., 105-106
Ge, X., 66, 68-69
Geertz, C., 53
Gibb, S., 40, 44
Glei, D. A., 18
Gonzales, N., 22, 68
Garbarino, J., 30
Gewirtz, J. L., 32
Gjerde, P. F., 65
Gollin, E. F., 35
Gottlieb, G., 32-33, 35, 61
Gottschalk, P., 96-97, 99
Greenberg, G., 27, 30, 33, 35, 61
Greenberger, E., 69
Greene, J. C., 130
Groginsky, S., 19, 58, 80
Guerney, V., 129

Habenstein, R. W., 51-53
Hagen, J. W., 40, 44
Hahn, A. B., 40, 58, 110
Hamburg, D. A., 6-8, 10, 58, 77, 110, 124, 126
Hannan, K., 22
Hanson, W., 68
Harold, R. D., 65
Harris, F. B., 106
Hartup, W. W., 34
Hawkins, J. D., 69
Hayer, C. D., 104
Heller, S., 51
Henry, W., 43
Hernandez, D. J., 3-12, 16, 30, 47, 56, 58, 70, 88, 96
Hetherington, E. M., 69, 70, 101-102

Hickey, T., 137-138
Hill, E. J., 67
Hill, J. P., 66, 68
Hill, M. S., 105
Hiraga, Y., 22, 68
Hirsch, J., 34, 86
Hoagwood, K., 138-139
Hofferth, S. L., 91
Hoffman, R. F., 28
Hofmann, S. D., 105
Hogan, R., 28
Holcomb, P. A., 80
Holmbeck, G. N., 66, 68
Homans, G. C., 34
Homes, C., 91
Hood, K. E., 34-35
Hoopfer, L. C., 84, 87, 106
Hops, H., 69
Howard, J., 29
Huang, L. N., 31
Huber-Yoder, M., 49
Hula, R. C., 32, 39, 127, 131
Hultsch, D.F., 137-138
Hunt, E., 69
Huston, A. C., 16-17, 19, 21, 109-110

Ignatiev, N., 51
Irby, M., 59
Irvin, C. E., 62
Itzkovitz, D., 51

Jackson, J. F., 40, 53
Jacobs, F. H., 87-89, 93
Jacobson, M. F., 51
Jacobvitz, D. F., 69
Jenkins, R., 30-31
Jensen, P. S., 138-139
Jessor, R., 75
Joebgen, A. M., 71
Johanson, P. C., 109
Johnson, B. L., 67
Johnson, C., 64, 69
Johnson, J. A., 28

Kagan, J., 27, 35-36
Kahn, A., 87

Kahn, R. L., 125, 129
Kamerman, S., 87
Kamin, L. J., 35
Kandel, D. B., 69
Kao, M., 69, 76
Katchadourian, H., 129
Kaufmann, M. B., 28
Keith, J., 70
Kendall, P. C., 38
Kenny, M. E., 67
Kerns, D., 75
Kerr, B., 69
Klerman, L. V., 18
Knight, B. P., 65
Knapp, J. R., 67
Knott, J. H., 32, 39, 127, 131
Kohn, L. P., 47
Kolaric, G. C., 71
Kondratas, A., 79
Kortlander, E., 38
Kossek, E. E., 49
Krampen, G., 66
Kretzmann, J. P., 44-46
Kuhn, T. S., 137
Kurdek, L. A., 70

Ladewski, B., 70
Lamberty, G., 30-31
Lamborn, S. D., 63-65
Larson, R. W., 66
Lee, V. E., 62, 70
Leffert, N., 114-115, 117, 121, 123-125
Lerner, J. V., 8, 28, 36, 49, 61, 70-71, 94, 129
Lerner, R. M., 1-4, 18, 21, 23, 25, 27-28, 30, 32-41, 43-44, 58-59, 61-64, 67, 71-73, 76-77, 81, 84, 87, 91, 94, 106, 117-118, 120-121, 127, 129-131, 136-137, 139-140
Lewontin, R. C., 35
Li, J., 15
Lightfoot, S. L., 22
Lindenberger, U., 25
Linney, K. D., 58, 80
Lipsitt, L., 39
Little, R. R., 117-118, 121, 128

Liu, H., 119-126
Lomax, R., 67
Lord, S. E., 66
Lorenz, K., 32, 34
Luster, T., 75, 114, 116

Macoby, E., 63, 70
Madison, T., 69
Maggs, J. L., 68, 70-71
Man, D., 119-126
Marteman, H. J., 103
Martin, J. A., 63, 105
Mason, C. A., 22, 68
Masters, R. D., 28
Matute-Bianchi, M. E., 22
McAdoo, H. P., 12, 20-21, 30-31, 28, 41, 43, 49, 53-57, 59, 114, 133-136
McCarthy, K. A., 66
McClelland, P., 37-38, 40, 133
McCubbin, H. I., 20-22
McGuire, S., 69
McKinney, M. H., 3, 4, 32, 37, 39, 58, 61, 62, 81, 91, 127, 131
McKnight, J. L., 44-46
McLanahan, S., 96-97, 99, 010-103, 105-106
McLoyd, V. C., 18, 21-22, 43
McNally, S., 66
Melby, J. N., 64
Meyers, M. K., 91
Mikulincer, M., 65
Miller, B. C., 67
Miller, J. R., 25, 39, 127, 131, 137
Millstein, S. G., 62
Mindel, C. H., 51-53
Modell, J., 30, 34-35
Moen, P., 37-38, 40, 133
Moffitt, H., 105
Moilanen, D. L., 67
Mont-Reynaud, R., 65
Moore, K., 18, 79-84, 101, 105, 110, 134
Morelli, G., 8, 19-20, 79-80, 88, 110
Morgan, M. C., 75
Morris, P., 25, 38, 133, 138
Morrison, D. R., 18, 101

Mounts, N., 63-64, 65
Muller, C., 71
Murray, C., 105
Murray, L., 119-126

Needle, R. H., 69-70
Neitman, P., 22
Nelson, C., 70
Nesselroade, J. R., 36
Nightingale, D. S., 80
Nisbet, R. A., 35
Novikoff, A. B., 27
Norton, M. C., 67

O'Leary, W., 124
Olson, H. C., 69
Ooms, T., 101-103
Ostrom, C. W., 130, 136-137
Overton, W. F., 32

Papini, D. R., 67
Parke, R. D., 30, 35, 44
Patterson, G. R., 68
Paul, B., 40, 44
Paulson, S. E., 64, 66
Petersen, A. C., 38
Peterson, L., 70
Peterson, P. L., 69
Philip, D. G., 47
Philips, D. A, 13, 88, 91-93, 107
Phinney, J. S., 45, 65
Piaget, J., 32, 33, 37, 129
Pieniadz, J., 66
Pike, A., 69
Pittman, K. J., 59, 111, 116, 119, 121, 125-126
Plomin, R., 32, 69
Primavera, J., 22

Ragsdale, E., 58, 107
Raley, R., 11
Ramirez, J., 45
Rathunde, K., 38
Reddy, M., 17
Reese, H. W., 36, 39
Renick, M. J., 103

Reiss, D., 69
Richards, M. H., 66, 71
Riegel, K. F., 28, 34
Roberts, D., 62
Robinson, W., 22
Roehlkepartain, E., 102
Roggman, L. A., 67
Roosa, M., 65
Roosevelt, W., 51-53
Rose, S., 35
Rosenbaum, E., 69
Rosenthal, D.A., 65, 75
Roth, J., 119-126
Rowe, D. C., 33-35, 37
Rubenstein, J. L., 68
Ruch-Ross, H. S., 22
Rueter, M. A., 66
Ruff, C.D., 39

Sahlins, M. D., 28
Sam, D. L., 65
Sameroff, A. J., 23
Sandefur, G. D., 96-97, 99, 102-103
Santrock, J., 69
Sargeant, M., 22
Savas, S. A., 22
Scales, P. C., 111, 113-117, 121, 123-125
Sears, H. A., 71
Sharma, A. R., 111, 113-116
Schaie, K. W., 129
Scharbach, J., 70
Schneirla, T. C., 28, 61
Schorr, L., 12, 18, 77, 81, 109, 119, 124, 127, 137
Scott-Jones, D., 75
Seiter, R., 69
Seltzer, J., 101-103
Shagle, S. C., 68
Shimizu, H., 65
Silverman, P., 119-126
Simmons, R. G., 129
Simon, L. A. K., 41, 134
Simons, J. M., 16, 17, 66
Simons, R. L., 64, 66, 68-69, 76
Small, S. A., 75

Smetana, J. G., 68-69
Smith, E. W., 81, 91
Smith, L. B., 23, 25, 33-34, 58, 80
Smith, R. S., 20
Smith, S. L., 19, 58, 79-84, 89-90, 90-91, 98-99, 110, 134
Smyer, M. A., 34
Snyder, N. O., 105
Spanier, G. B., 1-3, 63, 109, 129
Sparks, E., 128
Spencer, M. B., 20-22
Spenner, K. I., 4
Staudinger, U. M., 25
Steinberg, L., 63-65, 68
Stevenson, H. W., 64
Stice, E., 69
Stief, T., 81
Stingle, K. G., 32
Stoneman, Z., 67
Streissguth, A. P., 69
Sullivan, M. L., 76
Sweet, J., 10, 11

Taffel, S. M., 105
Taylor, R. D., 62, 69
Taylor Gibbs, J., 31
Terry, P. A., 3-4, 32, , 37, 39, 58, 61-62, 81, 127, 131
Thelen, E., 23, 25, 33-34
Thomas, A., 28, 36
Thompson, A. I., 22
Thompson, C. J., 70
Tildesley, E., 69
Tobach, E., 27-28, 30, 33-35, 61
Tout, K., 68, 79-84, 110, 134
Thomas, A., 129
Trickett, E., 138-139
Tryon, W. W., 40
Tsunematsu, N., 4
Tubman, J., 28, 35-36, 40, 130
Turner, R. A., 62

Vasquez García, H., 30-31
Ventura, S. J., 105
Verhoef, H., 8, 19-20, 79-80, 88, 110

Villarruel, F. A., 3-4, 37, 40, 53, 61-62, 81
Vinovskis, M. A., 105
Virden, L. M., 65
Wallerstein, J. S., 69, 102
Walsten, D., 34-35
Walter, B., 45
Wapner, S., 23, 33
Washburn, S. L., 28
Washienko, K. M., 45
Wasik, B. H., 30-31
Watkins-Ferrell, P., 22
Weinberger, D. A., 64, 68
Weiss, H. B., 124, 130
Weller, A., 65
Werner, E. E., 20, 30
Wethington, E., 37-38, 40, 133
Wetzel, J., 43
Whitbeck, L. B., 66, 69, 76
White, A. B., 75
Wierson, M., 70
Wilcox, B., 84, 87, 104-106
Wilson, L., 18, 21
Wilson, M. N., 47
Wolters, C., 40, 44
Wood, D. N., 64
Wright, D. W., 70
Wu, P., 69
Wulczyn, F., 4

Yang, A., 16, 17, 66, 68
Yau, J., 68
Yang, M. H., 67

Zabin, L. S., 75
Zaslow, M., 58, 69, 79-84, 88-91, 110, 134
Zeldin, S., 111, 116, 119-121, 125-126
Zigler, E., 41, 136
Zill, N., 81, 101
Zimiles, H., 62, 70
Zimmerman, M. A., 45, 62

Subject Index

Abortion
    in adolescence, 73
    poor women, 106
Academic policy, 130
Acculturation, 64
Adaptive modes
    among minority families, 21
Adolescent
    fathers, 73, 74
    pregnancy and childbearing, 72, 75, 105, 106
    sexual behaviors and problems, 72-75, 104-106
Adolescents
    as parents, 71-77
Advocacy groups, 135
Affirmative action, 52
African American children, 5, 8
African American families, 21, 54-57
    religion, 57
    stress absorbing systems in, 21
    structure and function, 55-57
    volunteerism, 56
African savannah, 28
AIDS, 72, 103
Aid to Families with Dependent Children (AFDC) program, 58, 79-81, 85, 89, 91, 93, 96, 97, 98, 100-102, 195, 110
Alan Guttmacher Institute, 73-74, 104
Annie E. Casey Foundation, 12-14
Applied Developmental Science, 41, 42
"Assets" maps of communities, 45-47
At-risk/poor children, stereotypes of, 109
Attachment theory, 32
Authoritarian parenting, 63
Authoritative parenting, 63

Behavior genetics, 32, 34
Boys and Girls Clubs, 71, 119
Bronfenbrenner, Urie
    contributions of, 132-133
Bureau of the Census, 13

Carnegie Corporation of New York, 3, 8-9, 58, 71-74, 119
Carnegie Council on Adolescent Development, 117-118
Center for Population Options, 105
Center for the Study of Social Policy, 14, 16-18, 70-71
Center for Youth Development and Policy Research, 120
Child and Dependent Care Tax Credit, 93
Child care, 8, 20
    influences of, 91-93
    job training programs, 92
    welfare reform, 91-93
Child Care and Development Block Grant, 92
Child-rearing styles
    in adolescence, 63-64
    types of, 63
Children of color, 3
Children's Defense Fund, 16, 58, 62, 73, 135
Chinese American youth, 65
Civil rights, 52
Civil society, 2, 109, 117, 118
Classism, 31
Cohabitation, 10-11
Committee on Ways and Means, 101
Community-based programs, 128
    youth development programs, 71, 119-125
Continuity-discontinuity issue, 35-36

Cost, Quality, and Child Care Outcomes
 Study Team, 91
Critical periods, 34

Day care, 39, 111
Deficit models
 of poor communities, 44-47
Demographics
 developmental, 4
Developmental assets, 111-116
 list of, 112-113
 promotion of, 111-116
Developmental contextualism, 23-42,
 47, 61, 62, 126, 140
 agenda for scholarship, 130-1342
 basic and applied research, 130
 developmental systems, 25-42, 128
 diversity, 30
 family and consumer sciences, 25
 features of, 27-32
 home economics, 25
 intervention, 31, 131-132
 outreach, 137
 plasticity, 25
 policy and program implications,
  23, 127-140
 relationism, 25, 26
Developmental systems
 research and application, 32, 37-41
Development-in-Context Evaluation
 (DICE) model, 130
Developmental transformations
 poverty, 129
Developmental transitions
 poverty, 129
Diversity
 dimension of, 40
 family policy, 48-50
 family functioning, 76
 family structure and function, 47
 policies and programs, 47-48
 poor communities, 44-47
 religion, 47
 research, 40-41
 sexual orientation, 47
 study of human development, 43

Divorce, 101
 child support payments, 102
Dynamic interactionism, 27, 28, 37

Earned Income Tax Credit (EITC), 95
Ecological validity, 137, 139
Ecological view of human development,
 26, 31, 38, 140
Efficacy research model of NIH, 138-139
Emergency Assistance (EA) program, 79
Empty nest, 129
Entitlement programs, 79-81
Ethnic diversity
 African American families, 54-57
Ethological theory, 32
Evolution, 35
Evolution
 human, 28
Explanatory research, 38, 39
Externalizing problems, 22, 68
External validity, 137, 139

Families
 dual earner, 3-6
 farm, 5-6
 functions of, 1-2, 62, 109
 historical perspectives, 1-12
 minority, 7
 revolutions in, 5-12
Family
 as a social institution, 2
 conflict, 67
 contemporary instances of, 4
 definition of, 2
 diversity and policy, 57-59
 diversity and role of ethnic variation
  in, 51-54
 evolution, 1, 2
 female heads-of-households, 97
 non-traditional, 3
 one-parent, 5-6
 positive child development, 2
 stereotypes about White, 3, 9-10
 temporal perspectives about
  diversity, 2
 violence, 50

Family Diversity and Family Policy

Family policy, 2
    children, 109
    civil society, 109
    diversity as a "double-edged sword", 49-51
Family structure, 2, 62
    cross-sectional and longitudinal views of, 3
Family Support Act (FSA), 85, 86, 92, 102
Fathers, 8, 69
    absent, 22
    employment patterns of, 9
Fertility rates
    among diverse groups, 43
Food stamps, 105
Foster care, 3
Formal operations, 129
Four-H (4-H), 71, 119
Fusion
    in developmental systems, 27, 33

Generalizability
    diversity, 36, 37
German youth, 66
Grandparents, 6, 8
Great Depression, 26
"Goodness of Fit" concept, 94, 119

Hernandez, Donald J.
    historical and contemporary variation in the family, 5-12
History
    temporality, 35-36
Historical change
    normative and non-normative events, 30
Historical events
    non-normative, 52
Holistic theories, 27
Household size, 7
Human capital, 81, 110

Identity crisis, 129
Indian Health Services, 19
Individuals
    as sources of their own development, 36
Industrial Revolution, 8
Internalizing problems, 68
International Youth Foundation, 128
Intervention research, 38
Immigrant groups, 9, 51-54, 64
Immigration and Nationality Act of 1965, 52, 53
Integrative levels, 27
Israeli youth, 65

Japanese American families, 65
Job Opportunities and Basic Skills Training (JOBS) program, 79

Kids Count, 17
Kinship support, 62

Latino parents, 47
Life course perspective, 25
Life events, 22, 38, 39
Little League, 119

Marital disruption, 39
Marriage
    cohabitation, 10
Maternal employment, 8, 39
    influences of, 70, 71
McAdoo, Harriette
    contributions of, 21, 133-135
Medicaid, 105
Mexican American families
    familism, 50
"Minority groups", 43

National Center for Children in Poverty, 14-15
National Commission on America's Urban Families, 103
National Institutes of Health (NIH), 138-139
National Longitudinal Study of Youth (NLSY), 18, 116
National Research Council, 119, 125-126

Nature-nurture issue, 32, 35
"Needs" maps of communities, 44, 45
New Chances Demonstration program, 89
Non-governmental organizations (NGOs), 124
Nuclear families, 3

Office of Hawaiian Affairs, 19-20
Office of Special Education, Department of Education, 43
Outreach, 135-139
    collaboration, 136, 137
    community empowerment, 137
    developmental contextualism, 137
    integration with research, 135-137
    research model of NIH, 137-139
"Ozzie and Harriet" families, 3, 9, 10, 56

Paradigm shifts, 137
Parent-child conflict, 68
Parent-child relationships
    in adolescence, 65-71
    influences of, 66-70
    negative, 67-70
    positive, 66-67
Parenting, 58
    child rearing styles of, 37, 62-64
    definition of, 61, 62
    of adolescents, 61-71, 76, 77
Parenting styles
    influences of, 63-64
Parents' education, 7
Peer groups, 39, 40
Permissive parenting, 63
    indulgent and neglectful instances of, 63
Personal Responsibility and Work Opportunity Reconciliation Act (PRWORA; P. L. 104-193), 79, 82-87, 100, 110
Plasticity, 33, 34, 38, 41, 76, 77
Policy
    design, delivery, and evaluation, 127-140

individual differences, 129, 130
need for diversity sensitivity, 19
Policies
    public, definition of, 2, 3
Poor communities
    diversity within, 44-47
Positive youth development
    "five Cs" of, 118
    programs promoting, 44-45
Poverty, 71, 125
    causes of, 94-96
    child, 3, 11, 12
        and families, 13-23
        and high school dropouts, 13
        and well-being, 13, 14
        incidence of, 13-17
        in United States and other industrialized nations, 14, 16
        variation across United States, 14, 15
    hard versus soft interpretations of, 94-96
    individual and family problems associated with, 17
    maternal risk factors, 17
    Native Americans, 19
    racial variation in, 16-19
    racism, 22
    risk factors associated with, 16, 18
    "rotten outcomes" of, 2, 81
    single-parent families, 16
    "spells", 97, 98
    welfare, 18, 19
Presidents' Summit, 117
Probabilistic epigenesis, 32, 33
Problem behaviors, 45
Progress
    concept of, 35
Protective factors, 22, 45
Psychoanalytic theory, 32
Puerto Rican children, 6, 31
Public policy and diversity, 43-59

"Racial" culture
    of Whites, 51
Racism, 22, 31, 125

Reductionism and mechanism
 theories involving, 32
Relationism and levels of integration,
 35, 35
Religiosity
 family, 66
Remarriage, 11
Resiliency, 20-23, 45
 among poor and minority families,
 20-23
 minority families, 21, 22
Risk
 success stories among at-risk
 families, 20, 21
Risk behaviors
 among youth, 58
Role strain, 70, 71

Scouting, 119
Search Institute, 111
Self-care in adolescence
 and parental work, 71
Sexism, 31
Sexual abuse, 75, 76
Siblings, 6, 7
Single-parent families, 39, 50, 70, 91,
 101
 adolescents, 62
 female heads-of-households, 9
 welfare-to-work, 49
Social capital, 81, 109
Social class, 4
Socialization, 64
 defined, 64
Social policy
 poverty, 125
 racism, 125
Social support
 convoys of, 125, 129
Sociobiology, 34
Sociogenic theories, 34
Stepparenting, 10, 11
Stereotypes
 diversity, 49, 50

Temporary Assistance to Needy Families
 (TANF) program, 79
Theory
 practicality, 41
Transitional Child Care programs, 93
United States Department of Commerce,
 6, 16, 18
United States Department of Health and
 Human Services, 73-74
University-community collaboration,
 138, 139
 "best practice" in, 139

Welfare dependence
 "onion" model of, 94-96
Welfare mothers
 "moral fitness", 104
 stereotypes of, 104
Welfare policy
 children and families, 84, 85, 97-
 107
 features of, 90, 91
 fertility behavior, 106
 history of, 81-87
 "make 'em suffer" strategy, 103,
 105
 multi-generational strategy for, 80,
 88-93
 types of individuals and families on
 welfare, 93-96
 two-generation approach to, 80, 89,
 90, 99, 107
Welfare recipients
 point-in-time estimates of, 94, 97
Welfare reform, 58
 child care, 91-93
 diversity, 79-107
 policy themes of, 87-107
 "undeserving poor", 86
Welfare "spells", 96-98
Welfare-to-work programs, 49, 82-85
Working poor families, 91

Youth development programs, 77
 collaboration, 124
 community based, 119-125

databases pertinent to, 122
definition of, 121
evaluation of effectiveness of, 121-126
principles and practices, 119-121
promotion of positive youth development, 124, 125

YMCA, 119

Youth policy, 109-126
absence of in United States, 58, 59
national model of, 117-119
positive development, 107, 116, 117
potential dimensions of, 116, 117
problems resulting from absence of, 110, 111